Manual of Community Paediatrics

To our teachers for enthusing us to take up community paediatrics; our colleagues, past and present, for making such a good team; and our families, for their patience and understanding.

For Churchill Livingstone:

Medical Editor: Lucy Gardner
Project Editor: Antonia Seymour
Copy Editor: Paul Singleton
Project Controller: Mark Sanderson
Page Make-up: Robert Ramage
Indexer: Nina Boyd

Manual of Community Paediatrics

Second Edition

Leon Polnay BSc MBBS FRCP DCH DObst RCOG
Reader in Child Health, Nottingham University; Honorary Consultant Community
Paediatrician, Nottingham Community Health NHS Trust, Nottingham, UK

Mitch Blair BSc MBBS FRCP MSc
Senior Lecturer in Community Paediatrics, Honorary Consultant Paediatrician
(Community), Nottingham, UK

Nick Horn BMedSci(Hons) BM BS DCH
Senior Clinical Medical Officer in Community Paediatrics, Ashford, Kent, UK

Dilip Nathan BMedSci(Hons) BMBS MRCP(UK)
Lecturer in Child Health, Honorary Senior Registrar, Queen's Medical Centre,
Nottingham, UK

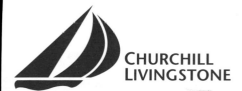

CHURCHILL
LIVINGSTONE

EDINBURGH LONDON NEW YORK PHILADELPHIA SYDNEY TORONTO 1996

CHURCHILL LIVINGSTONE
An imprint of Harcourt Brace and Company Limited

© Pearson Professional Limited 1996
except for growth charts © Child Growth Foundation 1994, 1995
© Harcourt Brace and Company Limited 1999

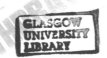 is a registered trademark of Harcourt Brace and Company
Limited.

First edition 1988
Second edition 1996
  Reprinted 1999

Note
Medical knowledge is constantly changing. As new information bcomes available,
changes in treatment, procedures, equipment and the use of drugs become necessary.
The authors and the publishers have, as far as it is possible, taken care to ensure that the
information given in this text is accurate and up to date. However, readrs are strongly
advised to confirm that the information, especially with regard to drug usage, complies
with latest legislation and standards of practice.

ISBN 0 443 05352 9

British Library Cataloguing in Publication Data
A catalogue record for this book is available from the British Library.

Library of Congress Cataloging in Publication Data
A catalog record for this book is available from the Library of Congress.

Printed in China
NPCC/02

The
publisher's
policy is to use
paper manufactured
from sustainable forests

Contents

5. Charts, tables and practical procedures   262

Preface

This handbook has been rewritten to take account of the rapidly changing state of our knowledge and practice since the first edition was published. Important changes have taken place in our child health surveillance programme, in immunisation, new growth standards and major organisational changes have taken place as a result of the 1989 Children Act and the 1993 Education Act.

Rapid progress has taken place with community child health becoming increasingly a secondary care service with family doctors mainly providing pre-school child health surveillance. The career structure for doctors has changed with closing of the career grades of clinical and senior clinical medical officer and opening of the staff grade and associate specialist posts. The training requirements of these posts and for consultants in community paediatrics are now well-defined.

A manual such as this cannot include details of the management of many individual conditions. This is the job of the heavier paediatric textbooks and of those of intermediate size such as *Community Paediatrics*, *Hospital Paediatrics* and *Essential Paediatrics* (all published by Churchill Livingstone) which are also written from Nottingham. The manual concentrates on the practical clinical systems in which this knowledge is applied. It is a navigational aid for those who are new to the framework of services in the community.

It is hoped that this manual will be of value to several groups: to family doctors as part of vocational training and continuing medical education, to trainees and established doctors in all branches of paediatrics, and to community nurses.

We have thoroughly revised all the original sections of the manual as well as adding several new sections, for example on practical procedures.

A manual of practice is as essential in the community as it is in the hospital ward, intensive care unit or outpatient clinic. It provides clinical guidelines for paediatricians and a description of the service to inform purchasers. We based the first edition of the manual upon our clinical practice in Nottingham so that it could form a framework for our whole clinical service and not just for individuals. Services should be constructed around the particular health needs of their population and there are bound to be areas where local practice differs from that recommended by us, because of the characteristics of the population. Local guidelines can also be more specific and well-used copies of the first edition often have additional local information, for example on referral pathways, written in the margin.

Revisiting the material in the manual is a humbling experience making one realise that the answer which might have once given a comfortable pass in an examination would now lead to a definite fail. We all need to question our own practice and recognise that education is not just the first part of our professional life, but all of it.

Thanks go to all our colleagues for providing the clinical environment in which this book was written. We acknowledge the direct and indirect contributions of all of the Nottingham paediatricians to this work.

Leon Polnay

Acknowledgements

The authors wish to acknowledge the following people and organisation: Ann Green, David Hull, Tom Hutchison, Eve Knight-Jones, Shirley Lewis, David Mellor, Eleanor More, Angus Nicoll, Connie Pullan, Wendy Rankin, Vidya Rao, Dianne Roden, Andrew Tandy, Ulla Trend, Jane Tresidder, Gareth Tudor-Williams, Helen Venning, Tam Fry and Child Growth Foundation for permission to reproduce growth charts.

1. PRINCIPLES AND ORGANIZATION

TEAMWORK

- The effectiveness of a community paediatrician rests upon teamwork with other professionals and partnership with parents
- The conditions necessary for good teamwork are:
  — Excellent communication
  — The ability to reach joint decisions
  — Knowledge of each other's professional skills and service organization
  — Continuity within each post
  — Personal and professional respect
  — A 'named person' coordinator, key worker for each family
  — Defined though flexible policies covering both inter- and intraprofessional organization, e.g. child protection procedures
  — Easy access to professional advice and support
  — Defined leadership and responsibility
- 'Liaison paediatrics' defines the important aspects of the specialty which do not involve patient contact but which ensure that all those who contribute towards an individual service plan work closely together

The community paediatric team

- This is the specialist paediatric team providing child health services to a defined community
- In an urban area, a team would cover a population of 100 000, approximately 20 000 children aged 0–15
- The team consists of:
  — Consultant community paediatrician (1–2 wte)
  — Doctors in training posts
  — Doctors in career posts – CMO, SCMO, staff grade, associate specialist
  — Community nurses
  — Administrative and clerical staff – an essential component
  — Local therapists
  — Attached social worker in a few teams
- Teams need:
  — A common base
  — A directory of local services

The roles of the team are:
- Prevention through:
  — Health education
  — Parent counselling
  — Immunization
  — Environmental changes
- Surveillance procedures leading to early diagnosis of:
  — Disorders of growth
  — Disorders of development: gross and fine motor, communication, vision, hearing, social, intellectual
  — Somatic disorders, dislocation of the hip, undescended testes
  — Emotional problems
  — Children experiencing emotional deprivation or abuse
  — Children experiencing physical or sexual abuse
  — Children likely to have special educational needs
- Management of:
  — Child-rearing problems, emotional and behavioural difficulties
  — Children with special needs, including special educational needs
  — Problems related to groups of children, for example in schools, day nurseries and family centres
  — General paediatric problems in conjunction with the family doctor or hospital paediatric services
- Advice to primary health care teams; teachers, educational psychologists; social workers and careers officers on children within the team's area
- Evaluation of the health and other needs of children within the team's area and the development of new programmes where current facilities are found to be inadequate (oversight of health)
- Teaching medical students, doctors, community nurses
- These roles are delivered through 14 programmes of care, each of which can be regarded as a contract

Services for all children

- Health promotion
- Accident prevention
- Core programme for child health surveillance
- Dental health
- Infectious disease control and immunization
- Adolescent health

Services for children in need

Social issues
- Child protection
- Children 'looked after'
- Adoption and fostering
- Disadvantage

Disability
- Developmental problems
- Emotional and behavioural problems
- Ill health (general paediatrics)
- Critical illness

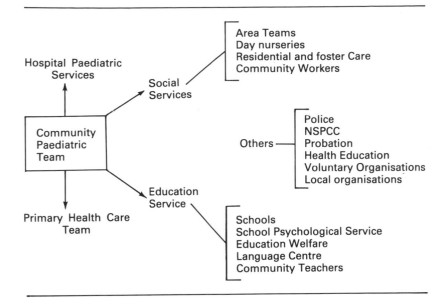

Fig. 1.1 Community paediatric team.

- Each of these programmes is provided by a *consortium* often involving many different parts of the health service as well as education and social services. This ensures that all aspects of a programme from prevention through to case-finding and management are fully integrated
- Within the team area the development of good local knowledge and working relationships with the other resources illustrated in Figure 1.1 is an essential component of successful work
- A locality profile and an annual report are means of identifying needs, disseminating information and identifying priority areas
- Each team can supply a specialist service to the whole district in a clinical specialty in which particular expertise is developed. Examples are learning disability; physical disability; hearing, speech and language problems; services to adolescents
- Within the team, there are named doctors and nurses for individual schools and clinics, with the intention of providing, as far as possible, continuity of care throughout childhood
- The team as a whole meets regularly to discuss current problems
- The teams within a district share common operational policies

RECORD KEEPING

- Types of record vary considerably between health authorities
- Familiarize yourself with their structure and format, and ascertain who is responsible for records 'upkeep' and storage so that a high standard of record keeping is maintained
- Notes may be used for:
  - Patient care
  - Collection of data for audit and research
  - Medico-legal reports
- Remember that what you write in the notes can be seen by other health professionals, court, parents and children (Access to Medical Records Act, 1991) so take care not to be inaccurate, libellous, flippant or insulting:
  - The following unacceptable examples are unfortunately genuine: 'small, dull, unattractive, bad-tempered child with...', and '...is getting uglier and uglier...'
- Good notes will be accurate, legible, concise and allow a 'story' to unfold about the child and his/her management
- A front sheet or summary sheet of main problems and management is useful

Each clinical note should consist of the following elements:
- Date
- Location child seen and type of clinic, e.g. school clinic, Radford or GP surgery
- Who was seen: child, parent, social worker, teacher
- How consultation arose, e.g. referral from teacher, school nurse, social worker, hospital team, primary health care team
- Reason for consultation – concern about vacant spells, growth, behaviour etc.
- History; include who from and how long
- Results of clinical examination and observation
- Summary of findings and your impression, e.g. withdrawn child with evidence of recent ear infection and residual glue ear
- Recommendations for investigation and treatment
- Advice and information given to parents/carers/teachers
- Follow-up arrangements, including where and when to be seen next and how long appointment should be – particularly important for clerical staff
- Identity of note writer – signature and name in print below this

Recent advances in records
- Parent-held and child-held records are increasingly used – not everyone feels at ease with this open system, especially where there are concerns about neglect and other forms of child abuse. It is important to discuss these issues with senior doctors
- Electronic records – using a computer on the doctor's desk. These

are not too far off and will make 'data entry' much more structured and easier to retrieve. Automatic coding of conditions (READ) is one advantage of this system

- Problem-orientated record keeping – a specific discipline using the notation SOAP: subjective, objective, assessment and plan

EQUIPMENT

Community paediatricians working in clinics, schools, family centres and in the home, need to have a portable 'kit' of equipment to take with them. The following is offered as a guide, though individual doctors will develop their own preferences. It is a compilation of equipment carried by individual community doctors in Nottingham.

Technical equipment
- Paediatric stethoscope
- Otoscope with insufflater (spare batteries); fibre-optic models give the best illumination
- Ophthalmoscope
- Thermometer
- Torch
- Magnifying glass
- Patella hammer
- Tuning fork (256Hz)
- Manchester rattle
- McCormick hearing test box
- Word lists and RNID speech discrimination test
- Eye occluder and fixation object
- Visual acuity charts for near and distant vision, e.g. Sonksen-Silver, Snellen, Stycar
- Red wool for vision testing at 6 weeks
- Colour vision test: Ishihara or City University
- Sphygmomanometer (paediatric cuff)
- Microtoise portable height measurer
- Peak flow meter

Support equipment
- Notepaper and envelopes
- Pathology and X-ray request forms
- List of important telephone numbers
- Dictating machine
- Growth charts:
  — Height, weight
    - Standard charts for population, separate charts for Down's syndrome
    - Preterm babies to 1 year of age
    - Velocity charts

- Body mass index
- Charts allowing for height of parents
- Boys and girls
— Head circumference charts
- Cole slide-rule calculator for height and weight
- Peak flow charts
- *British National Formulary*
- *Practical Immunisation Guide* and *Immunisation Against Infectious Disease*
- Height and weight conversion charts and/or pocket calculator (to imperial measurements)
- Star charts
- Small diaries for parents and children to keep records or for use in behaviour modification programmes
- Some key diagrams for explanations to parents and children, e.g. middle ear
- Frequently used health education materials

Developmental equipment
- Books, e.g. Ladybird *Talk About Home* and first picture books
- Symbolic toys, e.g. small male and female dolls, chair, spoon, cup, fork, dog, cat, car
- Crayons and paper with ready drawn shapes to copy
- Ten coloured one-inch cubes
  — To test block building, copying designs, matching colours, coordination
- Beads for threading
- Blunt scissors for testing fine motor skills
- Small jar with screw lid to test fine motor skills
- Access to standardized tests for those trained to use them, e.g. Griffiths, Denver, Schedule of Growing Skills

Bigger pieces of equipment for use in clinics
- Reliable weighing machine with a weight for standardization
- Stadiometer for accurate height measurement
- Sound level meter
- Audiometer
- Formboards, posting box and bigger toys

Sources of equipment
- Growth charts and measuring equipment:
  — Child Growth Foundation
    2 Mayfield Avenue
    London W4 1PW
- Manchester rattle:
  — Department of Audiology
    University of Manchester
- McCormick hearing testing kit:

- — Dr B McCormick
  Woodlands
  18 Nottingham Road
  Lowdham
  Nottingham
- RNID test:
  - — Royal National Institute for the Deaf
    28 Gower Street
    London WC1E 6AH
- Meg Warbler and sound level meter:
  - — Meg Instrumentation Ltd
    PO Box 32
    Sharrow Mills
    Ecclesall Road
    Sheffield S11 8PL
- Developmental testing equipment:
  - — NFER-Nelson
    Darville House
    2 Oxford Road East
    Windsor
    Berkshire SL4 1DF
- Vision testing:
  - — Clement Clark International
    Airmed House
    Edinburgh Way
    Harlow
    Essex CM20 ZED
  - — C Davis Keeler
    29 Marylebone Lane
    London W1
- Toys for developmental assessment:
  - — Most good toy shops
  - — Can also be ordered by catalogue from major suppliers, e.g.
    Nottingham Educational Supplies
    17 Ludlow Hill Road
    West Bridgford
    Nottingham NG2 6HD
- *Practical Guide to Immunisation in Children:*
  - — Julie Maltby
    Personnel Assistant
    Personnel and Development Directorate
    Nottingham Community Health NHS Trust
    Linden House
    261 Beechdale Road
    Aspley
    Nottingham
    NG8 3EY

(Information on Nottingham Video Training Packages, clinic records and parent-held records also available from this address)
- Personal child health record
  - Library held at:
    British Paediatric Association
    Royal College of Paediatrics and Child Health
    50 Hallam Street
    London W1N 6OE
  - Unistat
    Units 6/7 Bermondsey Trading Estate
    Rotherhithe New Road
    London SE16 3LL
  - Harlow Printing Ltd
    Maxwell House
    South Shields
    Tyne and Wear NE33 4PU
- *Immunisation Against Infectious Disease:*
  - HMSO Publications
    PO Box 276
    London SW8 5DT
    tel: 0171 873 9090
    fax: 0171 873 8200

PREMISES

Child health clinic and school clinic

Access
- Carefully situated with regard to public transport and main areas of population
- Ground-floor accommodation most suitable for access with young children
- Secure 'parking' necessary for prams and pushchairs
- Adequate car parking

Exterior
- Prominent sign to indicate the services available within

Reception area
- Signposted and prominent
- Welcoming

Waiting area
- Bright, spacious and comfortable
- Equipped with toys and books for children (a playgroup leader can work in this area; other activities, such as a toy library, can function at the same time as some clinics)

- Interesting, informative health education materials for parents, (pamphlets, wall displays, video)
- Toilets suitable for adults and children
- Space and privacy for changing nappies and feeding babies

Consulting rooms
- Comfortable and warm (22°C if young babies are to be examined)
- Quiet for confidential conversation; others unable to see in; secure from unintended interruptions
- If used for testing visual acuity, length of 6m necessary
- If used for hearing testing or speech therapy, should be sound attenuated
- Couch and screened off area to provide privacy for older children
- Chairs for adults and children as well as desk for doctor and low table for children
- Bins for disposal of nappies and 'sharps'
- Telephone (for communication, not interruption)
- Wash-hand basin
- Measuring equipment
- 'Childproof' cupboards

Treatment room
- Wash-hand basin
- Sterilizer
- Trolley
- Fridge for vaccines etc.
- Cupboards for storage

Storage space
- For records, equipment and supplies

School medical accommodation

NHS Act 1977 (Schedule 1) states that appropriate accommodation must be made available in schools for medical inspection.

Doctor's room
- Adequate size
- Adjacent hand-washing facility
- Reasonably quiet
- Privacy essential

Nurse's room
- Spacious enough for vision testing
- Height and weight equipment
- Hand washing facility
- Privacy

If schools are unable to provide this minimal standard, consider seeing individual children in a local community clinic instead. Parents and children will find it difficult to engage with a paediatric service delivered in a corner of a cloakroom or a store cupboard. Essential services within the school are discussions with individual teachers, which cannot easily take place in neighbourhood clinics.

CONDUCT OF A SESSION

When
- Essential not to clash with other clinics, school activities, bank holidays
- Availability of special educational needs coordinator for discussion
- Times to fit in with likely availability of parents
- It is a good idea when making a referral to find out when it is easiest to come and when impossible

Where
- Availability of required rooms
- Easy access and travel

Staff
- Availability of necessary medical, nursing and clerical staff
- Will you need an interpreter?

Records
- May need to be obtained from a variety of storage sites
- Very useful to read records of new referrals in advance; this helps if records are complicated; you are also able to anticipate what further information is required and request this ahead of the appointment

Appointment times
- You can also plan how long the appointment is likely to need and think about how you might structure the individual consultation. This can reduce the number of appointments needed
- If a very long appointment may be needed, make this the last in the session; this will mean that others are not kept waiting
- Remember that standards are set for waiting times, with a target of 90% being seen within 30 minutes of the appointment time

Referrals
- Referral letters may indicate urgency of referral and can usually give an indication of the length of appointment that is needed

Appointment letters
- Friendly, attractive and in simple English, giving place, time and directions, explaining what the appointment is for and what to do if they cannot come at that time
- A clinic pamphlet, explaining the service, who they are to see, what will happen, is very useful
- If you think there may be a problem with reading or with speaking English then a home visit or telephone call by clinic staff or a bilingual worker may be needed

Tools
- Availability of any special equipment, e.g. audiometer, stadiometer
- Venepuncture, investigation forms
- Charts

Room layout
- Plenty of chairs (adult and child)
- A low table, appropriate toys
- Move furniture so that family sit beside you, not with a desk as a barrier
- **If personal safety is likely to be a problem, make sure that you are not alone or can summon help quickly, and that the patient is not between you and the door. Fortunately such situations are rare**

Who: how many?
- At least 20 minutes for new referrals
- Usually 30–40 minutes
- Occasionally 1 hour
- Follow-ups 15–20 minutes
- Send appointments in good time; 10–14 days is usually about right, though some parents may ask for more notice
- Many child health clinics for pre-school child health surveillance do not have an appointment system because of the acknowledged difficulties of this with babies, and parents are asked to come on a particular afternoon. This type of clinic also has open access. The workload can, therefore vary widely

General: man's worst enemy is the telephone!
- Ensure that only essential calls are put through and that efficient messages are taken for the rest
- Tea or coffee are essential to survival
    — Find out the source and offer to pay
- Don't get lost!
    — A good map, directions and the address are also essential
- If you are running late, don't try to speed up to catch up. It is better to explain to each parent than to rush them through inadequately

Try to arrive a little early
- This enables you to check that everything is there and to receive information from nurses and teachers

Clinic record sheets
- Most services have some type of record sheet that needs to be filled in for each clinic to keep information, such as attenders, non-attenders, first appointment or follow-up, source of referral, GP, reason for consultation, time taken, outcome, who is conducting the clinic, date, place and type of clinic – this is for contracting purposes

- Remember to introduce yourself! It is much better to go outside and fetch and welcome the next patient than to ring a bell – the exercise will do you good and it helps *everyone* to feel more relaxed. Apologise if you are running late
- Ask for personal child health records
- Remember that listening to everyone is essential
- Explanations need to be repeated and can be written into the personal child health record. You can send the parents or the child a copy of the letter that you are sending to the GP
- Leave a little time at the end:
  — This is needed to discuss findings follow-up and to dictate letters
  — People don't like you rushing off
- When you leave, make sure that:
  — You have kept notes that need letters etc.
  — You have not left any important equipment
  — If the place is a mess from dropped biscuits, ground-in crisps or urine, apologise and let someone know
  — Say thank you and goodbye

HEALTH PROMOTION

- This will become an increasingly important sector of paediatrics as the prevalence of serious infectious diseases declines with successful immunization programmes while 'risk taking' behaviour contributes towards a larger proportion of both paediatric and, later, adult morbidity
- This should be a 'state of mind' and an intrinsic part of clinical practice
- It is also a team effort involving locality teams which have a common agenda, and a shared programme maintained over time
- Health promotion is now a major part of health policy in 'Health of the Nation' targets for coronary heart disease and stroke, mental illness, HIV and sexual health, cancer and accident prevention. Important individual areas for children and young people include smoking, alcohol, substance abuse, diet, obesity, teenage pregnancy, sexually transmitted diseases, accidents and self-harm. It is a major component of a district's public health policy and programme

There are three main approaches:
- Basic health education – the consultation
- Second-tier health promotion
- Third-tier health promotion

The consultation

Parents
- Accident prevention/smoking and appropriate nutritional advice

would be regarded as part of a normal consultation. Providing the advice without appearing patronising or overbearing is difficult. Improving knowledge alone can be insufficient in actually *changing* behaviour. Parents often establish their habits over years and, though aware of the medical consequences, are resistant to change, especially with other social pressures upon them

Suggestions
- 'Listening' to them
  — Establish clues about the family's perception of the problem. There are cultural variations between parts of Britain, let alone different ethnic backgrounds. Parents are influenced by financial considerations (e.g. cost of stair gates and car seats) together with 'powerful' figures within the family or supportive friends who guide the parents in daily child care

Advice
- Must suit the parents intellectually (without appearing patronising), socially and culturally
- Be specific, i.e. not 'stop smoking' but establish a programme. Stop over 2 weeks with a staged reduction
- May need to be seen over two or three consultations, even if the subsequent consultations are for unrelated problems
- Use multi-disciplinary support, i.e. health visitor/school nurse
- Research currently performed on audio/video-taped consultations suggests that this improves parental recall of consultations
- More impact if advice provided following a related illness, i.e. anti-smoking in a wheezy child or chronic otitis media
- Use leaflets with appropriate reading ages

Problems with implementation
- Time-consuming
  — Establish your own pattern of health promotion and start on the patients you have the best rapport with. Best way to experiment!
  — Focus the initial advice on one consultation, preferably soon after a related illness (see above)
  — Telephone support/follow-up is helpful in reducing the time you subsequently spend
- 'Becoming a nag!'

The child/teenager
- Similar to above, but please see sections on smoking/drugs/alcohol
- Most 'live for the here and now' so perceived future risks, i.e. lung cancer with smoking are not powerful indicators to stop. Tailor advice accordingly, i.e. smoking affects asthma/bad breath/and is expensive

Second-tier prevention

- Targeting large groups of people to improve health involves more organization and funding but is effective
- Advice may be obtained from your district health promotion department

The following scheme may be helpful:

Level one – identify need

- Identify the group
  — School children in a particular year or school/pre-school children to discuss diet, etc.
- Identify the need
  — Be clear about the areas you're targeting for health promotion. Dealing with all areas at any time can be a bottomless pit! Try to ensure that these 'areas of need' coincide with the children's/adults' needs too. They are more receptive if they feel it is relevant
  — Discuss with the rest of your team and obtain advice from local health promotion department or Director of Public Health
- Try to get baseline statistics
  — A simple questionnaire or 'brainstorming' session in a class/parent group can provide ideas on areas to be targeted. These pilot groups can be used to devise a survey of the entire group *before* intervention

Level two – organizing the programme

- There are many models of health promotion which suit different needs and groups

Suggestions

- Have clear aims – i.e. reduce prevalence of smoking/safe sex
- Education alone may be insufficient as the aim should be to alter the risk-taking behaviour
- Aim to empower the child/teenager/parent as opposed to developing a dependence on health professionals to guide them. This is significantly more effective and less time-consuming for health professionals
- Involve your whole team, primary health team or community paediatric team
- Develop 'health alliances'
  — This is advocated by the government and is more practical for busy health professionals. Local groups may already exist and teachers/day nursery staff and leisure services are usually interested in cooperating. It is important to work with them as opposed to 'taking over' because it is a health issue. This de-skills often competent staff, which detracts from the eventual need to empower the community

- Structure the programme with a timetable and clear definition of roles if involving multi-disciplinary staff. All involved parties should then receive copies of it (together with their managers/head-teachers) so as not to offend individuals
- Funding?
  — This may be included within existing contracts for health promotion
  — Alternatively, it may be necessary to apply for new or additional funding
    Local health investment programmes or joint finance with the local authority
    Charities
    Local industry – e.g. cinemas/supermarkets
    National bodies – research and development funding (will need to justify project with research aims and evaluation)
    If this is a research project, it may need ethical approval
- Most programmes need to be long term with 'intensive periods of education or intervention'. This 'immunization' model assumes that the change in behaviour will occur over a period of time and the group need background support, but concentrated periods of activity involving individual areas
- Evaluation
  — Extremely important if it is a research project, but equally important as feedback to both the group and workers involved. This may be objective, e.g. salivary cotinine for smokers and teenage pregnancy rates locally or reported changes, e.g. on questionnaires

These projects are effective, even allowing for the initial outlay of time by busy doctors/nurses, and at the least should improve interdisciplinary teamwork.

Third tier

Advocacy
- Health professionals carry authority on local committees, or nationally. National policies can be influenced by either individuals or health groups. 'Sleeping policeman' or speed humps influence mortality from road traffic accidents while tax on cigarettes reduces teenage smoking. Both are examples of legislation being more powerful than education in research studies

CONSENT AND CONFIDENTIALITY

Consent
- Parental consent is required before children can be seen, or for medical information to be given to third parties

- For emergency situations, and in some child protection cases, for example, where there is an assessment order, parental consent is not required
- The presence of parents is the most easy way of safeguarding consent
- For older children at school, signed consent at school entry is usually accepted as the parent opting into the whole school health programme, and individual consent for each school nurse review is generally not needed
- Signed consent forms need to take account of language and reading ability
- Children under the age of 16 who are of sufficient understanding can give or withold their own consent to examination or treatment

Confidentiality

- In general, disclosure of medical information should be on a 'need to know basis' and after discussion with parents
- It is good medical practice always to discuss with parents the need, for example, for schools acting *in loco parentis* to have essential medical information
- The welfare of the child is paramount, and this duty in the 1989 Children Act to act in children's interests will enable doctors to disclose information in the interests of the child
- In terms of confidentiality, the following advice is given for persons under 16: '*any competent young person, regardless of age, can independently seek medical advice and give valid consent to medical treatment and the duty of confidentiality owed to a person under 16 is as great to any other person*' (BMA guidance)

SERVICES FOR ADOLESCENTS

Characteristics

- Independent access, i.e. self-referral in school
- Access outside of school time and place, e.g. city-centre teenage drop-in clinic
- Offer of confidentiality, though, if consent granted, should communicate with GP
- Well publicized
- Non-judgmental

Provide

- Information
- Counselling
- Contraceptive advice and supplies

- **Emergency contraception**
  - **Within 72 hours of intercourse**
  - **Two tablets of a high-dose combined oral contraceptive**
  - **Followed by two tablets after 12 hours**
  - **See after 3 weeks to ensure treatment is successful and discuss contraception**
- Advice on sexually transmitted diseases and safer sex

PROFILES

- A 'profile' of a locality or school is a form of description of the health and social needs of children and families
- It is used to help plan services for a particular area by highlighting specific areas of need, e.g. a high prevalence of teenage pregnancy or unsupported mothers
- The form of a profile varies but might consist of the following items:
  - Age/sex structure – proportion of boys/girls in each age band
    Ethnic minority composition
    Family patterns – proportion of single parents
    Social class distribution
    Proportion of case load on benefits
    Local accident data
    Numbers of children on the child protection register
- School nurses and health visitors often collect this information during their contacts with families
- There is a trend to use the information for resource allocation of nursing staff as well as for highlighting particular programmes of care which should be considered for an area or school
- Community paediatricians may find the following data items useful in planning the skills and seniority of doctor required in a particular area:
  - Free school meal index (proportion of children in a school receiving free school meals)
  - The numbers of children on the CPR (Child Protection Register)
  - Numbers of children on the disability or special-needs register
  - Number of children not registered with GPs
  - Number of children registered with GPs who are not carrying out pre-school child-health surveillance
- Profile data can be augmented by the use of local census data (1991)
- Involvement of the local community in the production of a locality profile may result in local action, e.g. awareness of accident black spots leading to the development of traffic-calming schemes
- Geographical mapping of profile data can be a potent means of conveying areas of need

Recommended data set for locality profiles

Local profiles of schools, families of schools, practice populations or small communities should include information on:

Environment
- Location, boundaries, housing, transport, amenities, school buildings

Residents
- School and local population, socio-economic profiles, age/sex structure, unemployment rates, race, ethnic and cultural background, family patterns

Health status
- Mortality rates, morbidity rates, accident rates, health risks, permanent sickness and disability, hospital admissions, immunization uptake, uptake of child health surveillance, alcohol and drug dependency, health beliefs, children in need (1989 Children Act), known health problems in the school community, known psychological problems in the school community, children with learning difficulties, children on child-protection register

Service provision
- Hospital and community paediatric services, (staff, activities, resources, accommodation), general practitioner services, social services, voluntary community activities, education services, family planning services

CONTRACTS

- 1990 NHS Act – reforms included the purchaser–provider split
- Contracts produced by commissioners responsible for health needs assessment in the local population
- Contracts with providers up to publication of the manual are in terms of the number of face-to-face contacts made between health professionals and their patients (clients)
- A problem with this system is the emphasis on volume of children seen and not quality
- As community paediatrics moves from a routine surveillance service to more referral work the appointments tend to get longer and the number of children seen fewer
- The liaison work carried out between doctors and other agencies, e.g. social services and education, especially in the areas of child protection and the production of statements of special educational needs is not recognised in this system
- There is a move away from contacts as the currency of contracting to programmes of care for children, e.g. disability, children in need, child protection, surveillance, health promotion
- Quality aspects are being increasingly added to contracts with penalties if standards are not maintained, e.g. patient waiting times

2. THE CORE PROGRAMME

PRE-CONCEPTUAL PAEDIATRICS

The aim is to give parents the best possible chance of having a healthy infant. The risk factors for having an abnormal fetus or child include:

Infection
- Rubella in pregnancy can lead to blindness, cataracts, congenital heart disease and sensorineural deafness
- Other congenital infections include CMV and toxoplasmosis, hepatitis, herpes and HIV
- Primary preventive measures including health education and immunization against these diseases, where possible, as well as early detection of infection in pregnancy can prevent significant morbidity in the fetus or neonate
- The school health service has an important role in ensuring that all school girls are immunized against rubella. The MMR programme has helped to obtain immunity at an earlier age
- HIV awareness and safe sex practice are an important part of the health education programme in school

Alcohol
- Risk of fetal alcohol syndrome: intrauterine growth retardation, dysmorphic features and mental handicap
- Thresholds may be low, and so all alcohol should be avoided in pregnancy
- 33% of girls age 14–15 admit to drinking alcohol once a week or more

Smoking
- Cause of low birth-weight and most potent risk factor for sudden infant death syndrome (SIDS). Increased risk of later respiratory disease in the infant
- Smoking should be avoided if at all possible during pregnancy
- Smoking cessation programmes in a school or general practice setting are an important aid to the individual

Drugs
- Long-term medication should be reviewed before pregnancy and potential teratogenic drugs stopped or substituted
- The list of drugs to be avoided in pregnancy is long and is found in the *British National Formulary*. General advice is to take no drugs other than those prescribed

- Drug and substance abuse (marijuana, cocaine, heroin, glue, solvent aerosols) needs to be vigorously tackled by appropriate school-based awareness-raising initiatives
- 18% of girls age 14–15 have tried cannabis, 12% have tried solvents, and 8% have tried dance drugs

Phenylketonuria
- The offspring of women treated for this condition as children are at high risk of severe mental retardation unless low phenylalanine diet is resumed before conception

Chronic disorders
- Diabetes, heart disease, epilepsy, renal disease, hypertension – these pose special problems in management. Therefore, women should consult their physician before embarking upon pregnancy
- Some adolescents with the above conditions will be unaware of future implications for parenthood and may need careful guidance

Genetic risks
- These are increased if:
  — Either partner has a serious congenital malformation
  — A close relative has a serious congenital malformation
  — A previous child has a serious congenital malformation
  — A history of recurrent stillbirth or miscarriage
  — Consanguinity
- These couples require referral to the genetic counselling service. Advice may be given on the level of risk and the availability of antenatal diagnosis
- It is not unusual for adolescents to be unaware of the existence of significant genetic disease in the family, possibly through parental fears or ignorance, and the unwary doctor may need to tread carefully when making enquiries

General health
- Poor general health, particularly nutrition, may result in fetal growth retardation and deficiency states after birth
- Folate supplements are an important preventive measure against CNS malformations, especially spina bifida
- Congenital rickets has become less of a problem nowadays as a result of vitamin D fortification of foods, such as margarine and cereals
- A good diet and healthy living are an essential part of health education and preparation for parenthood
- Emotional stress may contribute to an adverse outcome in pregnancy, and stress reduction modification techniques may be useful for vulnerable adolescents

BIRTH NOTIFICATION

- Required by law within 36 hours of a live or stillbirth (UK)
- Notification made by birth attendant (usually midwife) to District Medical Officer or Director of Public Health
- Systems subject to local variation

Data collected
- Identity of mother – name, date-of-birth, address
- Baby – date and place of birth, birth-weight, address after discharge
- Details of pregnancy and delivery
- Presence of congenital abnormalities
- Condition of baby at birth, APGAR scores
- Name of mother's general practitioner
- Whether Guthrie test has been carried out

Increasingly, data collection is becoming computerized.

Actions taken
- Health visitor informed – birth visit (10 days)
- Name entered onto child register in child health office; this initiates surveillance and immunization procedures
- Notification of congenital abnormalities to Office of Population Censuses and Surveys (OPCS) on form SD56. Summary of statistics about congenital malformations ascertained in the first 10 days are compiled and fed back to health districts
- Copy to Registrar of Births for cross-checking with Registrations
- Statistics generated: numbers of births, local breakdown by Parish and Ward, place of birth (home or hospital), birth-rate, separate analysis of stillbirths
- The child health office keeps these local statistics, and trends in births in different parts of the health authority are observed and recorded

BIRTH REGISTRATION

- Statutory requirement in England and Wales since 1836
- Parents have a legal responsibility to register the births of their children within 6 weeks of birth (1874 Births and Deaths Registration Act)
- Both live births and stillbirths must be registered
- Registration is made by a parent at the local office of the Registrar of Births, Marriages and Deaths
- Some hospitals are offering this service on site

Data collected
- Name of child, sex, date and place of birth
- Mother's name, usual address, maiden name, place of birth, date of birth
- Father's name, occupation, place of birth

Actions taken
- Issue of birth certificate
- Issue of National Health Service number and card to enable registration with general practitioner
- Collection of national statistics through notification to Office of Population Censuses and Surveys
- Collection of local statistics
- Late registrations followed up after 6 weeks (less than 0.5%)

GENERAL NOTES ON HEALTH REVIEWS

- Every consultation is an opportunity for health promotion activity
- 33% of children are living in poverty in the UK – consider this when arranging follow-up appointments with families of limited means. Is the advice being given realistic, and does it take into consideration the family circumstances?
- Could the consultation take place over the phone as an alternative? Consider this option where a child is severely disabled and access to a clinic may be difficult
- Consider the intellectual abilities of the parents/carers when giving advice on management; 1 in 10 adults in the UK has significant reading and writing difficulties

Each consultation consists of the following parts:
- Review of past records
- History taking from parents and child
- Obtaining new information by observation and examination
- Producing a written record of the history and clinical findings
- Interpreting the findings, drawing conclusions about normal and abnormal features as well as defining areas of doubt
- Telling the parent and child of your findings and asking permission to give or ask for information from others, e.g teacher, health visitor
- Outcomes
  - See next routine appointment
  - Request investigations or obtain reports from other professionals
  - Send information to other professionals
  - Review before next routine appointment
  - Provide treatment/advice
  - Refer for more detailed assessment

Cautionary notes
- Parents' surveillance is continuous whereas ours is episodic
  - Parents are nearly always right
- Failure to complete a particular test does not necessarily mean that a child is unable to do it – he may be unwilling, frightened, shy, tired, ill, might not like you, or may be thinking about something else

- The child who is described as 'uncooperative' may be unable to perform the task. Careful follow-up is required. This title may mask general developmental delay, a specific deficit in the system under examination or a behaviour problem that warrants further assessment
- Always make allowance for prematurity in interpreting developmental data on young children
- Look at quality of performance as well as simple pass/fail criteria
  - The means by which children accomplish tasks may be more important than the final answer
- Observation is often more informative than the performance of standard tests
- Routine examinations can become 'reflex' activities in which individual variation is lost together with individual observation
- Many children with undoubted evidence of delay in development and neurological signs are found to have no impairment at later ages
- Assessment of milestones is a very crude procedure for examining a most complex process
- Social, cultural, environmental and family factors are more important than medical factors in determining the outcome in individual children
  - Thus the influence of social class and legitimacy is greater than that of birth-weight on later development and progress
- Listen to the child and see things from his viewpoint

Seeing the child at home or in the classroom may dramatically change our perception of him and his family.

HISTORY TAKING

Community orientation – particular features to concentrate on include:
- What has brought this problem to your attention at this particular time (the Balint approach)?
- What do other observers think the issues are, e.g. nursery nurses, teachers, social workers, foster carers, residential staff, hospital nurses etc?
- What help has been sought already from the GP or other members of the primary health care team?
- What advice has been sought from relatives, friends and other sources? This helps to determine what perceptions or mis-perceptions of the problem might exist
- Who else is involved in the care and management of the child? Use of a graphical representation ('professionogram') (Fig 2.1) is sometimes useful as a reference
- Consider the use made by families of voluntary agencies, helplines etc.

Professionogram

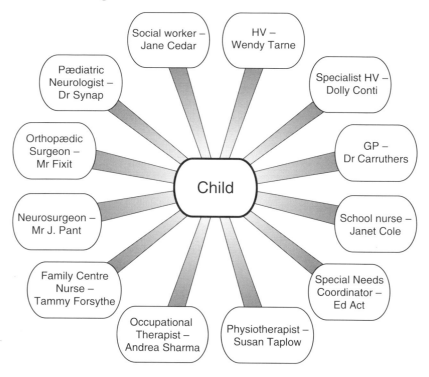

Fig. 2.1 Example of professionogram for a child of 4.5 years of age with spina bifida transferring to school.

- How does the problem affect the child's schooling, relationships with other children, or adults?
- Ask about activities of daily living: bathing, dressing, eating and toiletting
- Ask about leisure pursuits and hobbies and how any disability affects these activities
- Children smoke and drink alcohol – don't forget to ask about this
- Are the family receiving the benefits that they are entitled to, e.g. DLA, income support, invalidity care allowance etc?
- Family structure is very important to record accurately. There is nothing more embarrassing than addressing a step-parent by the incorrect surname or assuming that the woman that accompanies the child is the grandmother when it is the mother!
- One in four children are born out of wedlock. One in three marriages end in divorce. Use of 'genograms' (Fig 2.2) with standard notation should be encouraged as shorthand for a complex family structure

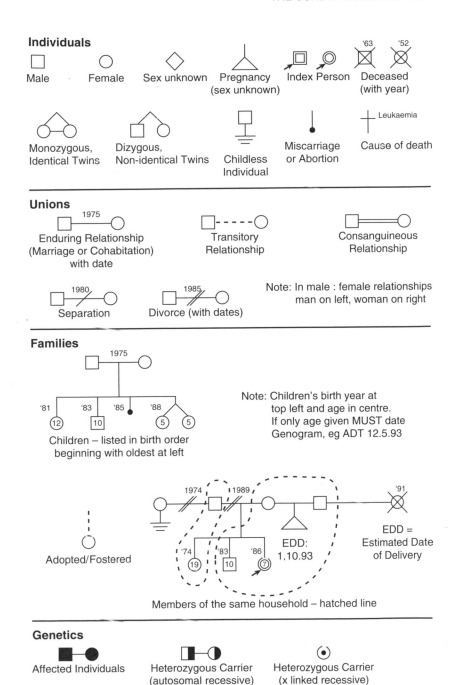

Fig. 2.2 Proposed universal genogram symbols. Genograms reproduced with permission from Tandy (1993, unpublished).

Physical examination
- Conditions in schools and certain settings may restrict the extent of examination
- Try and ensure that the child is seen in the most appropriate place for examination
- Privacy is essential and is a child's right
- The doctor should be sensitive to the needs of the child when others are present in the examination room, including nursing or medical students and friends of the child
- You must have an appropriate chaperone when the physical examination requires it

Some useful tips
- Take every opportunity to observe the child in different settings as this can often give more insight into how to manage a particular situation than in a purely clinic-based setting – a hemiplegic in the playground or a child with visual handicap in the gym
- Asking a child to write or read on the spot may give a false impression of poor performance. Ask the child or parent to bring you some school work previously prepared for you to look at
- It is no good examining a child's gait in a small examination room – a corridor is better and allows the child to run, which may accentuate physical findings, especially toe-walking and intoeing gait
- Holding an auroscope like a pen and resting your hand against the child's cheek stabilizes the ear piece and also reassures the child
- Talking to the child throughout and involving him or her in the examination is also very reassuring
- Ask children to undress themselves where possible both for dignity's sake and in dressing skills
- It is wise to record physical examination findings in the clinical notes as you go along so as not to forget essential information – this is especially important in child-protection cases
- With the younger child it is helpful to examine development on the floor, and a plain blanket or antenatal relaxation mat can be very useful to allow the child more freedom of movement than on a mother's lap

---

NOTES ON SURVEILLANCE PROGRAMMES

- 'Surveillance' is an engineering term applied to the checking of a product for defects – the term is falling out of favour as an umbrella term for all the activities involved in a *child health promotion programme*:
  - Early detection of impairment by screening (biochemical, sensory, physical examination, developmental, questionnaire)
  - Immunization

- — Health education
- — Health promotion
- — Monitoring of growth and development
- — Early treatment
- — Coordination of care
- — Support of parents and children
- Programme with checks at fixed ages safeguards children 'slipping' through the net, especially where there are frequent moves, changes of doctor or health visitor, or frequent medical contacts that allow attention on the known condition to overshadow screening for other problems
- The programme needs to be flexible because, in practice, the children are seen at a broad band of ages distributed around the 'landmarks'. Doctors and health visitors, therefore, should be able to make judgements about a child's development at any age
- Children who regularly do not attend the routine health reviews may be 'at risk' and should trigger a plan of action which might include home visits and gentle persuasion. Some parents are terrified themselves of injections and will avoid immunizing their children as a result
- The parent-held child health record is an integral part of the child health promotion programme and summarizes the reviews and health education messages. Try and familiarize yourself with the contents
- Notes on screening tests – the following criteria have to be met for a screening test to be employed (adapted from Hall and Michel). It is tempting to introduce new screening tests for aspects of child health surveillance, and checking against these criteria avoids unnecessary costs for both the health service and the family
  - — The condition is an important public health problem as judged by the value of early diagnosis in alleviating it
  - — There should be an acceptable treatment or other beneficial intervention for patients with the disease (occult or manifest)
  - — There should be facilities for diagnosis and treatment of the screened condition and these should be working effectively, i.e. there would be less value in early screening of hearing loss, for example, unless there was treatment available *soon* after testing
  - — There should be an early symptomatic or latent phase and the extent to which this can be recognised by carers and professionals should be known
  - — The test should be simple, valid, reasonably priced, repeatable in different circumstances, sensitive and specific and acceptable to the majority of the population
  - — The natural history of the condition and those that may mimic it should be known, e.g. neonatal jaundice due to biliary atresia, cf. breast milk jaundice

— There should be an agreed case definition of the condition and whether other conditions are likely to be picked up by the test and, if so, whether this is an advantage or disadvantage
— Treatment at the early, latent or presymptomatic phase should favourably influence prognosis or improve outcome for the family as a whole
— The cost of screening should be economically balanced in relation to the expenditure on the care and treatment of persons with the disorder and to medical care as a whole
— Screening as a continuous process, as opposed to a once-and-for-all project, needs to be justified explicitly

Pre-school child health promotion programme

General notes
- Each review consists of both screening and health promotion activities
- At each review, ask the parent for the parent-held child health record (PHR), read and review relevant sections, including parental observations, update the record in it and tear out any carbonless copies relevant to your service
- The PHR carries relevant health education material on nutrition, accident prevention, early recognition of illness, and dental health and you should use it to illustrate issues during individual reviews
- Children 'in need', including those who are the subject of abuse or neglect, are very often identified from the programme and you need to be aware of local child-protection procedures and referral contacts with local social services
- Coordination and supervision of the entire programme is part of the role of the District child health surveillance coordinator

Neonatal review

- This is usually carried out by the hospital SHO or, increasingly, by the GP or midwife if there has been a home delivery or short hospital stay

Review

Present pregnancy and delivery
- Risk factors include:
    - Complications of pregnancy
    - Birth asphyxia/low APGAR score
    - Low birth weight
    - Maternal illness and medication
    - Check results of early ultrasound scan

Family history
- Risk factors include:
    - Genetically determined disease, e.g. cystic fibrosis, sensorineural hearing loss, some causes of blindness, consanguinity

Social history
- Risk factors include:
  - Siblings in care
  - History of non-accidental injury
  - Young unsupported mother
  - Poor housing
  - Low income
  - History of parents having been in care or having been the victims of child abuse
  - Parental history of special education or psychiatric problems
- Presence of any of these factors may indicate the need for additional surveillance and support or the need to convene an urgent case conference where serious concern about the child exists

History
- History since birth from mother
  - Any worries about the baby?
  - Breast or bottle fed?
  - Any feeding problems?
  - Has baby passed urine and meconium?

New findings
- Baby is examined in the presence of mother

Observation
- General state of alertness or irritability, mother–child interaction, symmetry of movements, posture, abnormal facies, e.g. Down's syndrome

Colour
- Jaundice appearing within the first 24 hours requires urgent investigation
- Central cyanosis requires urgent investigation
- Peripheral cyanosis is generally not significant

Skin
- Neonatal urticaria – distinguished from skin sepsis by 'moving rash'
- Birth marks
  - 'Stork marks' very common and will fade
  - Strawberry naevi will increase in size for 1–2 years and then resolve
  - 'Port wine stains' remain static; on the face they may indicate intracranial problems, e.g. Sturge–Weber syndrome

Dysmorphic features
- Check for eye spacing, head shape, ears, mouth, skin creases, e.g. single palmar creases. Single features may be of little significance, but multiple features more strongly suggest a syndrome

Head
- Circumference <3 centile or >97 centile not always abnormal, but requires follow-up. Head circumference measurement in the

immediate postnatal period is notoriously inaccurate due to the fast rate of change in growth and scalp moulding
- Cephalohaematoma may take weeks to resolve and may lead to prolonged jaundice
- Sutures; wide sutures and fontanelle significant only if tense; absent or fused sutures need investigation/referral – this may cause asymmetry or abnormal contour

Mouth
- Exclude cleft palate and sub-mucous cleft by palpation. If present, refer to plastic surgeon

Ears
- Malformations of the face and pinna often associated with deafness; early audiological referral essential. Also association with urogenital anomalies
- Hearing should be tested in the high-risk neonate: premature, ototoxic drugs, family history, craniofacial anomalies
- Programmable oto-acoustic emissions (POEMS) or brainstem auditory evoked responses (BSAERs) are used for neonatal hearing screening

Eyes
- Look for abnormal movements, failure to fixate, opacities, absent red reflex, coloboma; if poor vision suspected, urgent ophthalmological referral required
- Profuse purulent discharge may indicate gonococcal infection requiring early treatment
- Rocking the baby gently over mother's shoulder is useful in causing the baby's eyes to open

CVS
- Look for central cyanosis, tachypnoea
- Palpate femoral pulses; precordium–heart size, thrill; liver size best indicator of failure
- Auscultation: soft ejection systolic murmurs are common and usually benign. If strong suspicion of congenital heart disease – refer. If slight suspicion in a well child – follow-up. Remember that even serious congenital heart disease can be 'silent'

RS
- Look for chest shape, tachypnoea and recession. Abnormal findings require investigation/treatment

Abdomen
- Look for distension – palpate for organomegaly; liver, spleen, kidneys normally palpable. Any abnormality requires investigation
- Umbilical herniae are common and generally resolve spontaneously
- A single umbilical artery may be associated with other congenital abnormalities
- Inguinal hernia; needs referral. May become irreducible and does not resolve spontaneously

Genitalia
- Testes: 10% undescended at birth (more if preterm). Should have descended by 1 year. Needs follow-up
- Penis: note position of meatus. Mild hypo- and epispadias easily missed. Needs referral
- Hydrocoele; common and generally resolves
- Ambiguous genitalia: require referral

Hips
- Test for instability by Barlow modification of Ortolani test. If abduction limited or hip dislocatable refer
- If all abnormal hips are to be identified, it is important to re-check hips at each visit until walking is established
- Ultrasound is increasingly being used for hip investigation or primary screening

Talipes
- If cannot be passively corrected – refer

Spine
- If scoliosis more than minimal – refer
- Mid-line abnormality may indicate underlying lesion
- Sacral dimple: if base not visible may be a sinus and requires referral. Dimple over the coccyx is common and does not have the same significance

Topics for health education at neonatal review
- Ensure that parents understand limitations of screening and that their observations are continuous as opposed to a 'one off' review examination and that they should return at *any time* to discuss concerns
- Advice on sleeping position – on back to avoid risk of cot death
- Advice on smoking cessation and effects of passive smoking
- Nutrition, baby care, sibling management, crying and sleeping problems
- Transport in cars

First two weeks – the birth visit

This is undertaken by the health visitor after the tenth day of life when she takes over responsibility from the midwife. It will often be her first contact with the family if there are no other children. An important objective is to establish a good relationship with the family.

Review
- The role of the health visitor and her place in the primary health care team
- Family's information about clinics, post-natal groups and other community resources
- Discuss the child health promotion policy and the records kept for each child, including the parent-held child health record
- Immunization to enable parents to make an informed decision

- General health of mother, her attitude to the baby, and reinforce the importance of the post-natal check
- Feeding patterns and problems
- Home conditions – material, social and economic

History
- Minor and major worries about child care, development, symptoms, signs, behaviour or general health
- Does mother think that the baby can hear?
- Does mother think that the baby can see?

Examination
- The extent of this is guided by the completeness of the neonatal examination and whether there are specific concerns

Topics for health education – first 2 weeks
- Nutrition and breast feeding, including peer support
- Smoking, accident prevention, bathtime safety, immunization
- Discussion of reasons for neonatal biochemical screening and the need for parents to request results
- Significance of prolonged jaundice
- Depression, and how to cope and obtain help

Review at 6–8 weeks

- Usually carried out by the GP or local community paediatrician – over 90% of GPs carry out child health surveillance on the children in their practice. Often combined with the post-natal check or immunizations
- In interpreting developmental and growth data, allowance must be made for gestation in pre-term infants

Review
- Information from birth notification and any discharge letters for babies from special care units or who are to have out-patient follow-up
- Family history and social history
  - Even though this information is often already available, it is better to go over it yourself, correcting errors and obtaining additional information that might not have been recorded in hospital letters
- Significance of social data may be seen more clearly in a community setting where local knowledge about housing and other family members may be most relevant

History
- Was this pregnancy planned?
- If not, did mother consider termination at any time or was she happy to continue with the pregnancy?
  - (These questions, if asked with sensitivity, often reveal important information about the mother's attitude towards the pregnancy)

- (For first babies): Have you looked after any babies before you had him?
  - Is it the same as you imagined, or different?
  - These questions often open up discussion about the unanticipated difficulties of parenthood
- If not the first baby, enquire about any difficulties in coping with more than one child
  - Ask about sibling jealousy
- What support or help is mother getting from husband, boyfriend, family or friends?
- Is she living on her own?
- Are there any financial or housing problems?
- Are there any worries about the baby that she wishes to discuss?
- Are there any problems with feeding? Is the baby breast or bottle fed?
- Is baby smiling?
- Does he look at mother and watch where she is going?
- Does he respond to her voice? (see clues list for hearing)
- How does mother feel herself?

New findings

Observation
- Is baby alert and interested in his surroundings?
  - If not, he is more likely to be hungry or sleepy than to have a serious problem
- Does baby dislike being handled?
  - This might indicate that handling at home is poor. The converse is also true, that a happy responsive baby is receiving very good care from his parents
  - However, an individual baby's personality has a big part to play independently of interactions with his parents
- Is the baby adequately clean and clothed?
- What is the quality of the mother's interaction with her baby? For example, warm, detached, seems depressed

Growth
- Plot all available measurements of weight, length and head circumference on a centile chart in the parent-held record and your own records if you are concerned
- Movements across centiles may indicate physiological adjustment or disease
- Careful history to determine that the child is receiving an adequate intake, and examination is necessary
- Investigation is necessary if downward drift continues without any explanation
  - Inadequate intake is the commonest cause

Colour
- Look for cyanosis and jaundice as in birth check

- Jaundice, if static, needs further investigation
- If breast-fed and fading, investigation is not needed, but follow-up is necessary to confirm this

Skin
- General inspection for seborrhoeic dermatitis, ichthyosis, ammoniacal dermatitis and monilia
- Strawberry naevi may have appeared since the birth check
- Mongolian blue spots are very common in children of Asian and African origin: they must not be confused with bruises

Head
- Measure head circumference and plot, checking growth since the birth check
- Look for tense fontanelles and upward shift across the centiles
- Plagiocephaly is common and resolves spontaneously

Dysmorphic features
- Look again for dysmorphic features
- Single features are probably not significant, but multiple features may indicate an abnormality

Mouth
- Check again for cleft palate
- Look for oral monilia: milk curds come off on the finger, monilia does not

Eyes
- Check red reflex (ophthalmoscope set to +6) to exclude cataracts
- Check that baby can fixate on an object 12" away and follow through an arc of 45° from the midline
- Look for nystagmus, manifest squint and structural abnormalities
- Any suspicion of poor vision requires urgent referral to an ophthalmologist
- Persistent clear or purulent effusion is usually due to a blocked naso-lacrimal duct; topical treatment with antibiotics may be required, with referral for probing if resolution does not occur by the age of 9 months

Ears
- Look again for abnormalities of the face and pinna as these may be associated with deafness
- If the parents suspect a hearing loss, do not delay referral until the 7 month hearing test

CVS
- See birth check
- Murmurs of congenital heart disease may have appeared since then

RS
- See birth check

Abdomen
- See birth check

Genitalia
- If testes are not descended, arrange referral

Hips
- Although universally examined at this age as part of the 6-week check, earlier examination is better to detect dislocatable hips and later examination (3 months) to detect the sign of limited abduction
- Continued surveillance is necessary until walking is established as not all will have physical signs early on
- Ultrasound, where available, may detect hip abnormalities in the absence of physical signs

Development
- See developmental summary charts (page 263)
- Look for asymmetry of movement and reflexes
  — Galant's reflex is particularly useful for this: with baby held in ventral suspension, stimulation of the skin down each side of the back results in flexion of the spine to the same side
- Look for apathy and lack of response
- Look for hypotonia and poor head control

Outcomes
- Normal growth, health and development
  — Congratulate parents
- Minimal deviation from normal
  — Explain to parents and arrange to review at or before next routine check
- Parental concern, but no abnormal findings on examination
  — Arrange to review at or before next routine check
- Unequivocal departure from normal
  — Explain and refer for more detailed assessment
  — Many children fall into an intermediate category and it may be wise to observe the rate of development for a longer period of time before referral
- Make sure that the GP and health visitor are aware of the findings and any special follow-up arrangements

Topics for health education – 6–8 weeks
- Immunization, nutrition, danger of fires (consider purchase or loan of fireguard), bathtime safety, avoidance of scalds
- Recognition of early illness, simple management of fever and advice on contacting the GP

Review at 2–4 months
- Re-check hips for limited abduction and other signs of dislocation (not all Districts carry out this policy)
- Immunization advice on local reactions and treatment
- Weighing of child as necessary

Review at 6–9 months

- Often carried out at time of distraction hearing test, usually by the health visitor

Review
- Previously identified problems
  - New information?
  - better/worse?
  - referral?
  - discussion?
- Changes of address, employment, family structure
- Changes in service provision
- Immunization
- Surveillance programme with parents

New findings

History
- Do parents have any problems that they wish to discuss?
- Is there any information they would like about general care, child development or local resources? It is usually useful to discuss these both before examination of the baby and as a 'running commentary' to one's examination, explaining what one is doing and the significance of any findings

Examination
Development:
- Discuss development (gross motor, fine motor, language, social), using the four charts in the appendix)
- Ask for parents' comments on each of the developmental items as well as recording your own observations
- Decide whether, on the basis of information collected, that all areas of development are within normal limits or define areas of uncertainty
- For marginal problems review in 1–2 months
- For greater problems refer for more detailed evaluation at clinic level

Hearing:
- Has baby passed hearing test? (see hearing section)
- If failed, what action has been taken?
- Do parents suspect any hearing problems?
- If not tested, arrange as soon as possible

Squint:
- Refer to ophthalmologist if:
  - Manifest or latent squint is present (see vision section)
  - Parents or others suspect one, even if not evident at the time of examination

Hips:
- Can also be checked at 3 months
- If both hips do not abduct fully, consider CDH or cerebral palsy

- Refer for orthopaedic or neurological opinion
- For CDH refer by telephone for urgent opinion
- Some babies have benign asymmetry with limitation of hip abduction, rib flattening and plagiocephaly – if in doubt X-ray

Growth:
- Measure weight, length, head circumference and plot on a centile chart, allowing for prematurity
- Compare with previous records
- Refer/investigate abnormalities (see growth section)

Topics for health education (6–9 months)
- Accident prevention: choking; scalds and burns; falls; bath safety – NOTE increased mobility – discuss safety gates, guards, car transport safety, buggy safety
- Dental prophylaxis
- Developmental needs
- Avoidance of sunburn

Review at 18–24 months

This review is usually carried out by a health visitor, either at home or in the clinic setting. Some health visitors carry out this review in a group setting.

Review
- Previously identified problems
- Changes of address, employment, family structure
- Changes in service provision
- Immunization
- Important life events – social and medical
- Surveillance programme with parents – development, child care, resources

New findings

History
- Do parents have any problems related to health, development or behaviour that they wish to discuss?

General review of development
- Progress reviewed with parents using charts and PHR
- Ask parents about language and speech development – use of formal tests can sometimes help parents to understand the nature of any delay in this area and the need for referral for further assessment
- Child should be using gestures appropriately and demonstrating clear communication skills with others, even if there are few words

Squint
- Suspected or confirmed squint should be referred

Non-walkers
- All non-walkers at this age should be seen by a doctor

- Most will be normal – bottom-shufflers or familial pattern
- CPK estimation should be done on non-walking boys at 18 months to detect Duchenne muscular dystrophy – important genetic implications of an early diagnosis
- Spastic diplegia may not be obvious until this age
- May be a marker to look for other features of developmental delay

Growth
- Height should be measured at this age. If review done on postal or telephone basis, then ensure that height has been measured opportunistically in the surgery
- Plot and compare with previous readings, allowing for prematurity

Topics for health education
- Accidents; falls from heights including windows, drowning, poisoning, road safety
- Behaviour – difficulties are the norm. Parents need advice on maintaining sanity and guiding behaviour in acceptable directions
- Teeth cleaning and use of fluoride supplements
- Developmental guidance on play, encouraging language development

Review at 3.25–3.5 years

This is a 'school readiness' review aimed at identifying any growth, developmental or behaviour difficulties which may need to be addressed before school entry.
- It is carried out by either doctor or health visitor and can be arranged at the time of the pre-school booster (3 years from primary immunization)
- The 1993 Education Act requires that the health authority notify the education authority if it believes that a child has or is likely to have any special educational problems or needs
- Although the majority of children with special needs will have been identified by previous reviews, this is an opportunity to review the case load to determine whether there are children who may have 'fallen through the net' – e.g. persistent non-attenders, non-immunized, those not in any nursery facility or with child minders
- Children who are identified as having special needs should be referred to the educational psychologist or to an appropriate pre-school discussion forum, e.g. DHT

Review
- Previously identified problems
- Changes in address, employment, family structure
- Changes in service provision
    - Is child attending nursery school or playgroup?
    - If not, are there any plans for this?
- Important life events – social and medical
- Immunizations up to date?
- This review is a good opportunity to introduce parents to the school health system

New findings

History
- Do parents have any concerns about health, development, that they wish to discuss?
- If at playgroup or nursery school, do the staff have any concerns about the child?

General review of development
- Progress reviewed with parents (and nursery staff) using developmental charts and PHR
- Observations by parents and others at this age will provide a much more complete picture of development than would formal 'testing'
- Watching a group of nursery children at play will provide good information on the very important developments in social interaction that occur at this age
- Gross motor and fine motor skills vary widely at this age. Children exhibiting difficulties in these areas will benefit from assessment and specific help (e.g. OT)
- Poor language development is the most reliable indicator of potential educational problems
    — These children require thorough assessment of general development hearing, and speech therapy advice (see language section page 96)
- If there are parental or professional concerns about vision, it should be possible to measure visual acuity using the Stycar single letter chart or, preferably, the linear Egan–Calver chart or Snellen letters matched to the Stycar key card (see vision section: page 102)
- Squint or suspected squint should be referred to an ophthalmologist
- Hearing: should be tested if concerned and you are adequately trained; otherwise you should refer

Growth
- Height and weight
- Plot and compare with previous measurements

Topics for health education
- Accidents: fires, roads, drowning
- Road awareness
- Playgroup/nursery – preparation for school
- Nutrition and dental care

SCHOOL ENTRANT REVIEW

School nurse

When
- First year of full-time schooling
- Age 5–5.5 years
- This will consist of a health appraisal by the school nurse

- In a few schools, where there is an exceptionally high level of need or very poor uptake of the pre-school child health surveillance programme, there is an argument for the school doctor seeing every child
- 1 in 5 children will have some form of special need at some stage in their education

By whom
- School nurse
- Selective referral to school doctor

Why
- To identify problems which may influence the child's general wellbeing, health or education
  - These may be in the areas of:
    Physical health
    Development
    Behaviour
    Social disadvantage (children in need)
- To meet the parents and introduce the school health service
- To give, with parents' consent, relevant information and explanations to the teaching staff

Time needed
- 20–30 minutes

Preparation
- Collection of pre-school records and checking that no parts are missing. For children born in other districts, transfer of notes must be requested. For many children, the pre-school information will be in the Personal Child Health Record, with non-carbonated copies being held by the clinic.
  - This task is carried out by the child health clerical staff and the school nurse
- Check records for:
  - Identified problems (development, health, behaviour)
  - Immunization status
  - Completion of pre-school checks
- Discuss with health visitor
- Find out any concerns of reception class teacher
- Invitation to parents emphasising the importance attached to their attendance and participation

School nurse health appraisal
- Explains content of school health programme and obtains written consent from parents
- General observation: skin, expression, demeanour
- Measurement of height and weight and charted
- Observation of posture and gait
- Measurement of visual acuity preferably using Snellen chart at 6 m, or by Sheridan–Gardiner if this is not possible
- Audiometry: performed by audiometrician or school nurse

Review with parents
- Previously identified problems
- Changes of address and employment
  — Many changes of address may indicate social problems and an unstable pre-school experience
  — Unemployment may produce severe social disadvantage
  — Employment: it is always useful to know which parents are doctors, nurses, teachers, psychologists, social workers etc. – ask for parents' occupations
- Family composition and history
  — Are other children all living at home (in care?)
  — What schools do the other children attend?
  — Identify those with special educational needs
- What other health professionals, if any, are involved?
- Recent visits to the GP
- Immunization status
- Any medication, especially if required at school
- Parental concerns: ask specifically about
  — Vision
  — Hearing
  — Speech (in mother tongue if appropriate)
  — Behaviour: settling into school; sleep; making friends
  — General health: absence from school; diet; energy
  — Any other parental concerns, personal or family problems that the parent would rather discuss on their own

Health promotion topics may include
- Diet
- Exercise
- General hygiene
- Dental heath
- Accident prevention
- Adjustment to school

Outcomes
- Continue with standard core programme alone
- Refer to school doctor or GP
- Referral to eye clinic
- Discussion, with parental permission, of relevant medical information with class teacher

Table 2.1 Summary chart of recommended core programme for school age child

Age	Clinical programme	Immunization
	School nurse	
5 years (year 1)	Structured school-entrant health interview conducted with parent	By age 5 a full course of DT, pertussis, polio, Hib and MMR should have been completed
	Height and weight Check completion of pre-school checks of heart, testes, pre-school concerns Visual acuity Hearing (sweep test)	
	Discussion with teachers to identify any concerns	
7–8 years (year 3)	*Paediatrician* Selective referrals from school nurse, taking account of teacher and parental concerns *School nurse* Visual acuity (Height and weight)[a]	
11–12 years (year 7)	Opportunity for general health check[b] *School nurse* Visual acuity Colour vision	BCG
14 years (year 10)	Opportunity for general health check[b] *School nurse* General health check Questionnaire to parents and pupils	
14/15 years (year 11)		Dip/T/polio

[a]Height at age 7–8 is indicated (a) where there is concern about the child's health or growth, (b) where there is incomplete or missing data for the pre-school years (i.e. less than three measurements between 2 and 5 years), and (c) children whose height at 5 is on or below the -2 SD line (2nd centile).
[b]More detailed health checks at these ages are required for the individual where there is concern expressed by the child, parents, teacher or from health records; or for the population where school profiles indicate high levels of deprivation or other special circumstances.

School doctor (selective)

There is a *menu* of items, so that all or a single relevant aspect of examination may be included. This depends upon the reason for referral.

History (see section on paediatric history taking)
- Information from school nurse health appraisal
- Information from reception class teacher
- Full medical history
  - Family history (genogram)
  - List of professionals involved (professionogram)
  - Social history
  - Past medical history
  - Developmental history

Examination (general appearance and behaviour, observed during history-taking)

Appearance
- Cleanliness/neglected/tired?

Behaviour
- Is he shy towards the examiner?

Demeanour
- Does he relax during the examination or remain clinging?
- Is he constantly on the move?
- Is he easily distracted or does he have good concentration?
- How does he interact with his mother?
- Is there evidence of conduct disorder?
- Frozen watchfulness? Consider child-protection issues

Parents
- Do they appear in good health?
- Do they appear tired, depressed, anxious, aggressive, apathetic?
- Did parents have any difficulties when they were at school? – e.g. literacy

Development
- Assessment may be included where parents, teachers, or the school nurse are concerned

Hearing
- Review history and audiometry results
- Inspect tympanic membranes
- If audiometry results doubtful, perform speech discrimination or McCormick toy discrimination test
- Refer children with significant losses for investigation, ENT management or to Children's Hearing Assessment Centre for those with suspected severe problems
- Children with borderline problems may be kept under observation in school or school clinic
- Criteria for referral must include many factors, such as language development, general concentration and ability, mother tongue other than English

See hearing section for a full discussion (page 88).

Language
- Observation: young children are often inhibited, and language is often best observed from spontaneous utterances while history-taking
  — Try taking the family history from the child!
  — If asked the names of brothers and sisters and whether they are good or naughty, many children will produce long, complex and interesting accounts
  — Parents may totally silence their children by commanding them to *'speak for the doctor!'*
  — Also beware the parent who says 'of course he understands everything I tell him'
- Spontaneous: he should produce sentences of 4+ words, with appropriate word order and few omissions, correct use of past and present tenses
- Pictures (e.g. Ladybird *Talk About Home* book)
  — Often useful if spontaneous speech is not heard
  — Should be able to name colours, explain simple picture sequence, name fruits, find parts of the body on animal or doll, answer 'what could we put in here?' (milk bottle or carton), 'could mummy sit on this?' (holly) Why not?
- Record:
  — Articulation problems
  — Comprehension problems
  — Expression problems
- Refer to speech therapist if there are problems, discuss with teacher
  — Arrange review if problems borderline

See language section for a fuller discussion (page 96).

Fine motor skills
- Teachers will generally report if there are any problems
- If there are no concerns, it is usually adequate to observe the child drawing a picture of mummy while notes are being written up
  — This should include head, trunk, legs, arms, eyes, nose and mouth. If trunk absent, details such as eye lashes, pupils, fingers acceptable
- If concern expressed, look for:
  — Immature pencil grip
  — Incoordination
  — Tremor
  — Involuntary and associated movements
- Useful activities in which to test these are:
  — Copying square (90–95% are able to)
  — Copying triangle (80% are able to)
  — Building a tower of 10 bricks
  — Building steps of bricks

Gross motor skills
- Probably not necessary to test formally in all children
- Teachers and parents well able to identify which children are less skilled at PE, are much slower than others at gross motor tasks, fall frequently, or are poorly coordinated
- If concern expressed, look for:
  - Abnormal gait – uneven or broad-based
  - Abnormal posture on standing
  - Arms stretched above head: look for signs of hemiparesis or dystonic movements
  - Stand on one leg (8 secs 90%)
  - Hop (5+ hops)
- If concern about gross motor skills is confirmed, then a full neurological examination is necessary

Vision
- 6/6—6/6   repeat at age 8
- 6/12+   refer
- Unequal vision less severe than 6/12   retest
  - Deteriorated to 6/12   refer
  - 6/6—6/9   repeat at age 8
  - 6/9—6/9   repeat at age 8
- Squint   refer
- Nystagmus   refer
- Movements not full   refer

See vision section for a full discussion (page 102).

Physical examination

Growth
- Plot height and weight on percentile chart
- Record parental heights
- Compare with previous records of growth
- Consider referral if:
  - Below 0.4th centile or above 99.6th centile
  - Crossing one complete channel between measurements
  - Below 2nd centile with tall or average parents
- If borderline repeat height and weight in 3–6 months
- Most problems can be sorted out at local level by clinical examination, accurate height and weight velocities, parental heights, and bone age

See growth section for a full discussion (page 123).

Face
- Normal appearance?
- Dysmorphic features?
- Is the child anaemic, jaundiced or cyanosed?

Skin
- Check for eczema

- Infections
- Suspicious injuries
- Abnormal pigmentation

Teeth
- Are they clean and healthy?

Throat
- Are tonsils healthy?
- Lymphadenopathy?

Ears
- Examine tympanic membranes
- Dull? Retracted? Perforations?

Heart
- Is there a murmur?
- If there is, check pulses, cardiac impulse, and BP
- 97th centiles for BP
    — 3 years 112/78; 6 years 116/79; 9 years 125/85; 12 years 135/87
    — BP should not be used as a screening test, but should be
      included as part of full examination of the cardiovascular
      system where this is indicated
    — Height related centiles are also available (see section 5).
- Soft ejection systolic murmurs limited to the LSE are benign and
  very common (50% of children)
- Pathology is suggested by a diastolic murmur, thrill, abnormal
  peripheral pulses, radiation to the neck, abnormal heart sounds,
  symptoms, e.g. SOB, general signs, e.g. clubbing or cyanosis,
  abnormal ECG or CXR

Chest
- Note shape, symmetry, respiratory rate and movements
- If abnormal, or if there are symptoms, auscultate

Spine
- Observe the spine in the standing position for scoliosis
- Look for any associated asymmetry of the chest, e.g. rib hump
- Postural curves disappear when the child bends forwards
- All others require further assessment
    — Progressive curves and those greater than 10–15 degrees
      require referral
- Trials are currently taking place to assess the value of school
  screening programmes for scoliosis; at present this is not
  recommended as a screening test

Abdomen
- Palpate for enlargement of liver and spleen or masses (many school
  medical examinations are carried out in rooms that do not have
  couches – only gross abnormalities can be excluded by examination
  in the standing position)
- Check hernial orifices
- Are both testes in the scrotum?

- Review previous records
- If not in the scrotum, are they retractile?
- Retractile testes descend when the child squats
- Refer all others
- Is the foreskin non-retractile?
  - Most will after gentle retraction in the bath
  - History of balanitis, ballooning during micturition or a very narrow orifice on protraction indicate the need to refer for circumcision

Legs

The following problems may be identified:
- Flat feet
  - Only rigid or painful feet need referral
  - Examine the arch when the child is on tip-toe
- Intoeing
  - This may be due to metatarsus varus, medial tibial torsion or femoral anteversion
  - Most will resolve spontaneously
  - Children with rigid joints, neurological signs, suspected rickets or Blount's disease (sharp angulation below the knee) need referral
- Knock knees
  - Most will correct spontaneously, but an intermalleolar distance greater than 10 cm indicates that this is less likely and the child should be referred

See orthopaedic section for a fuller discussion (page 159).

Outcomes

Explain to parent
- Child is healthy, his development is normal
  - Routine surveillance by school nurse
  - Doctor will see again if parents, nurse or teachers request it
- Child requires follow-up/observation, or further investigation by the school doctor
  - Explain when and why
- Referral is necessary, e.g.
  - General practitioner
  - Speech therapist
  - Educational psychologist
  - Social worker
  - Another paediatrician
- Medical referrals must be discussed with the GP
- Ask permission to discuss relevant problems with the child's teachers and encourage parents to do the same
- It is useful to give parents and teachers a written account of important information

— In many Districts this is incorporated into a parent-held child health record
- 10–20% of children will have a problem needing follow-up or treatment

SCHOOL HEALTH APPOINTMENTS AFTER THE SCHOOL ENTRANT REVIEW

Paediatric appointments

Following the review of all children at school entry, a selected group will be followed-up by the doctor either within the school as part of his regular visits or in a school clinic serving a group of schools. These consist of children with special educational needs in cooperation with the special educational needs coordinator, Children in Need and children where monitoring on management of health or behaviour problems in school is desirable. Other children will be referred at later ages at the request of the school, by referral from the family doctor, or because of parent or pupil concerns.

Although the Education Authority has a duty to provide appropriate accommodation within the school, the school clinic, which is often in a Health Centre, will provide better facilities for further examination, investigation and management.

The following problems should prompt a referral to or discussion with the school doctor:
- Persistent ill health
- Children who are sent home on more than one occasion because of ill health
- Children who spend more than the occasional time out of the classroom on medical grounds
- Persistent school absence
- Increasing behaviour problems
- Academic failure
- Marked incompetence in physical activities
- Signs of neglect or abuse
- Social problems

Review is often valuable, especially for children with special needs or those who are known to respond poorly to change, when they move to a new school. A parental and/or pupil questionnaire is often used to accompany the core programme to identify *new* problems or parental or pupil concerns. General and open-ended questions and reference to the personal child-health record are much better than a list of yes/no enquiries about specific conditions.

Review at 14 years (year 10)
Aims
- To ensure that the school leaver and his parents fully understand the significance of past and present medical problems

- To discuss with them the possible effects of medical problems upon training and employment
- To enlist, where necessary, the services of the careers officers or specialist careers' officers for those with special needs

Selection for referral to the school doctor; this is done at a 'conference' on the basis of the following information:
- Parent questionnaire
- Pupil questionnaires, or
- Joint parent/pupil questionnaire
- Information from school medical records
- Information from school nurse
- Information from teachers
- School doctor, nurse and senior teacher are usually all involved in the selection

Procedure
- Review identified problems
- Investigate any new problems
- Ask about career intentions
- General advice
  — Many school leavers confuse prospective employers by giving inaccurate or irrelevant medical information, e.g. febrile convulsions or other conditions completely resolved may be confused with current problems
- Specific advice:
  — Some medical conditions may preclude certain occupations
  — It is necessary to consider the intended career and possible effects of the condition under the following headings:
    Is the young person unsuitable for work which requires accurate vision?
    Is the young person unsuitable for work which requires accurate colour vision? This would include many jobs in the armed services, police, airline pilots, bus and train drivers and some jobs in industry requiring accurate colour matching
    Is the young person unsuitable for work requiring accurate hearing?
    Is the young person unsuitable for work out of doors exposed to bad weather? e.g. children with asthma and other chest and heart problems
    Is the young person unsuitable for work in a dusty atmosphere? e.g. asthma
    Is the young person unsuitable for work involving a lot of prolonged standing or walking? e.g. children with motor handicaps
    Is the young person unsuitable for work at heights? e.g. children with epilepsy and vestibular problems
    Is the young person unsuitable for work involving moving

machinery? e.g. children with poor fine motor skills
Is the young person unsuitable for work involving handling
wet materials – water, oil, chemicals? e.g. many skin
conditions

- Although this is a list of prohibitions, it is important to be positive
rather than negative
- This list is only a guide, and consideration must be given to the
degree of difficulty that the child will experience within any given
category
- Problems such as transport to work, mobility within the workplace,
intellectual and emotional factors need to be considered
- Careers officers (and the Employment Medical Advisory Service)
need accurate and sometimes detailed medical information to
complement their knowledge of specific occupations

For children leaving school, especially those with special needs, a
summary report to the young person and family with a copy to the
family doctor can be very useful.

The school nurse

- The school nurse may be attached to a number of schools or may
work full time in a single large secondary school or special school
- She will see all children for health appraisal on a regular basis
throughout their school years
- In the UK she can see children and examine them without prior
parental consent, in contrast to the doctor, where consent is
needed. However, it is recommended good practice to obtain
parental consent to opt into the school health core programme and
to respect the right, in the Children Act 1989, of children and
young people of sufficient understanding to give or withhold
consent

Roles of the school nurse

Health appraisal
- This involves:
  — Screening by history, observation, examination and
    measurement (see table of core programme: page 42)
  — Collating information from school staff
  — Affords opportunities for individual counselling and health
    education

Core programme
- Carried out at 7–8 years
            11–12 years
            14 years
- Review of known problems
  — Progress in school

— Any difficulties or worries that the child may have. The nurse usually knows the children very well, and children may often bring personal problems to her

Referral because of new problems
- These may come from parents or pupils, teachers, the family doctor or the community paediatrician
- Appointment could include consideration of:
  — Reason for referral
  — History related to illness, absence from school, major changes in the family
  — General care and cleanliness
  — Emotional state, e.g. withdrawn, depressed, tired, extrovert, aggressive, evasive, immature, 'odd'
  — General development
  — Monitoring of height and weight: measured and plotted
  — Vision and hearing testing where there are relevant concerns
  — Skin conditions, including bruising
  — Condition of hands and feet
  — Hair and scalp
  — Posture and gait
  — Mouth: oral hygiene and dental caries

Outcomes
- Continue with standard core programme alone
- Offer health advice to parents and pupil
- Offer, with parental permission, health advice to the school
- Follow-up or referral as a child in need
- Refer to school doctor or GP
- Other referral, e.g. eye clinic, teenage clinic

Liaison functions
The school nurse has a central role in providing continuity of knowledge and care for individual children and liaison with others.
These may be:
- Parents through home visiting
- School doctors
- Health visitors
- Teachers
- Social workers and education welfare officers (*Children in Need*)
- Speech therapists
- Audiometricians
- Physiotherapists and occupational therapists
- Clerical staff of the Child Health Unit

Management functions
These may include:
- This will form part of a health care plan at school
- Collaboration is vital with teachers, the primary health care team and the community paediatrician

- Supervision of medication in school
- Supervision of other forms of treatment in school, in special schools or for pupils with special needs in ordinary schools
- Treatment of enuresis with doctor
- Advice on diet, including obesity and poor diets on an individual or group basis
- Monitoring medical problems, e.g. peak flows in asthma; growth; vision; hearing; skin problems
- Health advice and health education activities in cooperation with school doctor and teachers (pastoral care staff and health education coordinators)
- Arranging treatment of minor skin and hair infections and injuries

Other roles of the school doctor and nurse

The school doctor and nurse are not just visitors who come 'and do the medicals' without any other contact or knowledge about the school. In order to be useful, they need to know how the school is organized, the stresses and problems within the school, and the nature of the environment (social, cultural and physical) from which the children come. A School Health Profile will give a picture of this and the main health problems and needs within the school. This can form the basis of an annual report to governors and the Director of Public Health, which contains specific recommendations for action.

They need to know:
- The members of staff and what their special roles may be within the school
  — Special educational needs coordinator
  — Child protection coordinator
  — Teachers with pastoral care responsibility
- The programme for health education within the school, and to be available, where necessary, to advise or participate

They may need to advise on:
- General health matters within the school
- Endemic problems such as solvent abuse, non-accidental injury, bullying, sexual abuse and sexual assault, tattooing, healthy eating, control of infection

They may need to speak to:
- Parents' groups
- Teachers' groups
- Children's groups, e.g. classes, clubs, various project work, careers days

They must be able to communicate:
- They need conditions of privacy, warmth and reasonable comfort to carry out these tasks effectively
- Good secretarial and clerical help are the other essential components

3. SPECIAL NEEDS

NEONATAL FOLLOW-UP

The follow-up of survivors of neonatal intensive care is increasingly regarded as mandatory; although there are no precise health service guidelines, there is considerable consensus on how it should be done.

Reasons for follow-up
- To identify children with disability at the earliest stage and give all possible help to the child and family
- To audit usefulness of neonatal intensive care and its cost in terms of disability
- To assess trends over time and make comparisons between units
- To understand the epidemiology of disability

Which children should be the subject of special follow-up?
- Very low birth weight infants – BW less than 1500 g – prevalence of disability in this group is 18–25% in published studies
- Gestation less than 29 weeks – prevalence of disability 23%
- Hypoxic ischaemic encephalopathy. Preceded by central nervous system depression at birth as assessed by an APGAR score of less than 6. One-third of this group is liable to have significant disability
- Survivors of meningitis, hydrocephalus, intraventricular haemorrhage associated with persistent parenchymal echodensities and/or ventricular dilatation on ultrasound
- Seizures (with or without encephalopathy)

Programme for follow-up
- Some children will need to continue to attend a neonatal follow-up clinic in hospital because of continuing need for medical treatment
- Others will be discharged well into the community; these children require
  — 100% uptake of routine child health surveillance programme by an experienced practitioner
  — Additional tests of vision by an experienced ophthalmologist to detect retinopathy of prematurity and neonatal hearing screening
  — Referral into a child development centre for full assessment programme for those children causing concern

Child health clinic or opportunistic contacts
The doctor in a busy clinic is faced with a child who was previously

discharged from the neonatal clinic or lost to follow-up. The following guidelines may be useful:

- Most severe cerebral palsy is identified by 1 year, and moderate cerebral palsy by 2 years
- Specific learning and physical disabilities may become apparent only later in otherwise normal school children
- Behaviour problems are commoner

Plan

- Enquire about specific problems. Motor clumsiness, numeracy and writing delay and lower reading ages are a few possible outcomes which will not be identified on routine developmental screening (i.e. Denver test) and require specific tests, i.e. Griffith assessment or Stott – Moyes – Henderson test of motor impairment. May need referral to educational psychologist, community paediatrician
- Check with local neonatal follow-up scheme
- Behaviour problems may need referral to a clinical psychologist (see behaviour section)
- Assess cerebral palsy as in previous section
- Be aware that the pre-term infant born in September will have the added burden of starting school 1 year ahead of peers regardless of degree of prematurity and its coincident problems

Research/audit/data collection

The volume and depth of information is variable, depending on local needs. Minimum criteria include:

- Definition of disability – local or national guideline followed
- Mortality following discharge from the neonatal unit needs to be recorded as it is increased often due to broncho-pulmonary dysplasia or sudden infant death
- Cerebral palsy (prevalence in very low birth weight children 7.5–10.5%)
- Severe cognitive impairment – DQ less than 50 (2–5% in very low birth weight) (Moderate cognitive impairment – DQ 50–70 is included by some but is a more variable finding, less constant over time than severe cognitive impairment.)
- Hearing impairment
  — Moderate threshold 40–70 db
  — Severe 70–90 db
  — Profound over 90 db
- Visual impairment
  — Corrected visual acuity less than 6/24
- Epilepsy requiring treatment
- Hydrocephalus requiring a shunt
- Behaviour problems may be included but are less easy to assess unless a standard questionnaire is used
- It is necessary to record how many children have multiple impairments

- To know the causation of the disability is helpful, e.g. intracranial haemorrhage
- Non-neurological sequelae include prolonged oxygen requirement due to broncho-pulmonary dysplasia; growth less than 3rd centile; severe scarring, limb amputation, tracheostomy, stoma or short gut or bowel problem, chronic renal failure

Method of assessment
- Age – 2 year/4 year and 8 year if possible
  - Detailed neurodevelopmental assessment (i.e. Griffith scales) by experienced paediatrician
  - Sociodemographic information (i.e. parental occupational, maternal education and social support status)
  - Perinatal data
    CRIB score (index of severity at neonatal unit admission)
    Duration of stay + or – respiratory assistance and cranial ultrasound findings

The effect of a premature birth date on the timing of a child's education
Nowadays increasing numbers of very premature children survive and enter mainstream education. There is no reason to suppose that being born early leads to an early maturation of the child's brain or its abilities. A child who is due to be born in September, and who comes into the world 12 weeks early, will, in addition to all the problems already mentioned, be obliged to enter school a whole year early, go through the whole of his or her education a year early, including public examinations. This is an additional disadvantage, leading to stress and poor achievement. It seems only logical for these children to have their educational entry and leaving dates calculated from their date of expected delivery.

CHILDREN IN NEED

The Children Act 1989
A child is defined by the Act as being *in need* if:
- He is unlikely to achieve or maintain, or to have the opportunity of achieving or maintaining, a *reasonable* standard of health or development without the provision for him of services by the local authority

- His health or development is likely to be significantly impaired, or further impaired, without the provision

- He is disabled, i.e. 'deaf, dumb, blind or suffers from mental disorder of any kind or is substantially or permanently handicapped by illness, injury or congenital deformity or such other disability as may be prescribed'

Duties of the local authority include:
- To identify the extent of children in need
- To provide services to support families with children in need, including day care, respite care, family aids, counselling and accommodation
- To prevent neglect and abuse
- To publish information about services
- To maintain a register of children with disabilities

Duties of the health authority include:
- Identification and referral of children in need
- To cooperate with the social services department
- To contribute towards assessment and review

Children 'looked after'
- Children provided with residential care under the 1989 Children Act are called children 'looked after'
- The local authority has a duty to enhance the quality of life of children living away from home and to provide aftercare
- Backgrounds include family breakdown, abuse and neglect
- Problems include discontinuity in health care, poor uptake of preventative health care, poor compliance with treatment, school non-attendance, learning difficulties, conduct disorders, self-harm, substance abuse, teenage pregnancy, prostitution and sexually transmitted diseases
- Require targeting of community child health services

THE CHILD WITH SPECIAL NEEDS

- There is no universally accepted language of disability, and terminology may be confusing. The terms 'special needs', 'disability', 'disablement', 'handicap', 'normal', 'disadvantaged' may be interpreted differently by different individuals, groups or professions
- Disability may be viewed according to various models, e.g. medical, social, religious
- For statutory purposes, special educational needs are clearly defined in the 1993 Education Act
- The following definitions were proposed by the World Health Organization in the International Classification of Impairment, Disabilities and Handicap (ICIDH 1980), in the context of health experience:
  — *Impairment.* Any loss or abnormality of psychological, physiological or anatomical structure or function
  — *Disability.* Any restriction or lack (resulting from impairment) of ability to perform an activity in the manner, or within the range, considered normal for a human being
  — *Handicap.* A disadvantage for an individual, resulting from an

impairment or a disability, that limits or prevents the fulfilment of a role that is normal (depending on age, sex or cultural factors) for that individual

Disease or disorder → impairment → disability → handicap

Example
In spina bifida, the lesion itself is the impairment, and inability to walk is the disability. The handicap will depend upon the age of the individual, being quite different for a school-leaver than for an infant

Aims of services for children with special needs
- Cooperation with child/young person and parents/carers
- Prevention – by optimal prenatal, perinatal and postnatal care
- Early detection of impairment
- Early intervention
- Easy access of services
- Optimal provision of services
  - Health
  - Education
  - Social services
  - Voluntary
- Ongoing support for child and family and continuity of care

SERVICES FOR THE CHILD WITH SPECIAL NEEDS AND HIS FAMILY

The community paediatrician has an important role in coordinating the integration of services. He or she therefore needs to know the basic provision from health, education and social services. Details will vary locally, and can be found in local handbooks produced by the various departments. This information also needs to be kept up to date with changes in personnel and practices. The service needs to be robust and very well coordinated between age groups (pre-school, primary and secondary age, further education and services for young adults) and between assessment centres and locality schools, clinics and primary health care teams.

Health service provision

District handicap teams and assessment centres
These provide a coordinating function within a district for the assessment of children with complex special needs. Handicap teams and assessment centres may form a single organization or may be separate, but with very close links. Similar assessment facilities may be provided on a more local (patch) basis within a district according to resources. The functions are:
- Investigation and assessment of children with complex disorders:

— This is a multidisciplinary assessment which may involve any
of the following disciplines, depending upon local
arrangements:
    Community paediatrician
    Hospital paediatrician
    Paediatric neurologist
    Specialist nurses
    Orthopaedic surgeon
    Ophthalmologist
    Audiologist
    Psychiatrist
    Clinical geneticist
    Psychologist
    Educational psychologist
    Teacher
    Physiotherapist
    Occupational therapist
    Speech therapist
    Social worker
— Assessment, which is completed over a number of days, is
followed by a 'case conference' to correlate information,
discussion of results with parents, and the production of a
written report
— The written report contains a summary of the assessment
findings, including diagnosis, and recommendations on
treatment and follow-up; it is circulated to all relevant people
— Many centres also provide a written report for parents
— The assessment may provide the basis for medical advice for
statutory assessments of special educational need
— Registration on a special needs/disability register may follow
— Initial assessment leads on to a programme of management
based on its recommendations; each recommendation will
have a series of objectives to be achieved; review
appointments will monitor progress and achievement of those
objectives and a series of new recommendations and
objectives are set. Reviews may be carried out as a repeat of
the initial assessment procedure, but confined to the smaller
number of professionals who are directly involved
— Many centres identify a key worker for each child; this worker
is a named point of contact with the centre; it is good practice
to ensure that the key worker choice is approved of by the
parents as an individual with whom they feel comfortable
• To arrange and coordinate treatment:
    — This may be provided in a hospital-based assessment centre,
    at school, in a day nursery, at home or in hospital or
    community clinics
• To provide advice and support to parents and child-care staff

- To liaise with local voluntary organizations
- To link with district services for learning disabled
- To act as an information source within the district on childhood disability
- To organize seminars and courses of training for professional staff
- To be involved in epidemiological surveys of need
- To monitor the effectiveness of the district service for disabled children
- To present data and suggestions for the development of the service

Community paediatrician
- Provides support and advice to children/young person and parents/carers
- Coordinates the management of children with special needs within the community, working closely with other professions
- May be a member or chairman of multidisciplinary assessment team/district handicap teams
- Provides medical advice on children with special needs who attend mainstream school or special units
- Provides medical advice to special schools and day nurseries
- Provides medical advice to specialist careers officers
- Acts as a source of advice on children with special needs within the community

General practitioner
- Provides continuity of care for whole family
- Manages general health needs
- Prescribes continuing medication

Health visitor and specialist health visitor
- Provides advice and support within the home for the pre-school handicapped child
- May provide advice and support to other family members
- May have an important coordinating role, particularly with GP
- Specialist health visitors can provide an important resource of knowledge and expertise to their colleagues as well as to parents

Education service provision
Educational psychologist
- Provides advice to teachers in mainstream schools on the management of children with special educational needs
- Provides advice to parents of children with special educational needs
- Coordinates statutory assessments of special educational need
- Works closely with school medical services

Pre-school service – e.g. parent-teacher counsellor, portage worker
- Provides assessment, advice and support at home to parents of children with special needs prior to school placement
- Liaises with LEA on child's possible future educational needs

Peripatetic specialist teachers
- Provide advice and support to teaching staff on children with special needs who are placed in mainstream schools, e.g. children with hearing or vision problems
- Support pre-school children with sensory impairments, and advise their families

Specialist careers officers
- Receive medical reports on disabled school leavers and advise on:
  — Courses of further education
  — Work orientation and work experience courses
  — Direct or sheltered employment
  — Non-vocational courses, e.g. social and leisure skills
  — Employment rehabilitation schemes
  — Day units

Social service provision
- The following may be provided:
  — Social work support and casework
  — Day care
  — Residential care
  — Respite care
  — Financial help and advice
  — Advice on housing and adaptations
  — Main agency for learning disability after school leaving
- Provide assessment under the Disabled Person's Act 1986 to ensure a smooth transition for a disabled child between full time education and adult life
- Required under Children Act 1989 to maintain a register of children in need, including children with disability

Recreation and holidays
- Schemes may be available from a variety of sources:
  — Voluntary organizations
  — Self-help groups
  — Social service departments
  — Leisure service departments
  — Education departments

Limits of service provision
- These are determined by:
  — Cost
  — Local policy and legislation
  — Access
      Geography
      Transport
      Mobility
  — Wishes of the child and family

SPECIAL NEEDS STATISTICS

- 20% of the school population will at some stage in their education have some form of special educational need
- 4% of children aged 0–4 years, 6% of children 5–15 years and 7% of young people 16–19 years have limiting long-standing illness reducing their functional capacity
- In 1991 one-fifth of young people of 16–19 years reported long-standing illness – mainly asthma, skin disease and ear disease
- Prevalence of chronic illness in childhood has doubled between 1972 and 1991
- About 2% of children attend special schools – varies widely across the country, depending on the availability of resources and local educational policy
- Severe learning disability, SLD (IQ < 50) occurred in 3.4 per 100 live births in England and Wales in the early 1980s prior to prenatal screening
- The most common single causes of SLD are Down's syndrome, cerebral palsy, spina bifida and X-linked disorders

At birth
2.5–3% have a congenital abnormality (figures per 10 000 total births of selected anomalies):

Foot deformities: 15.4
Urogenital: 12.3
Cleft lip and palate: 11.7
Cardiovascular: 8.6
Down's syndrome: 5.9
Central nervous system: 5.1

- Rates of serious congenital anomalies reported soon after birth have remained constant over the past 10 years with the exception of CNS anomalies, which have reduced
- Congenital anomalies are more common in infants of mothers born in Pakistan – risk factors include high fertility, consanguinous marriages and cultural and religious objections to prenatal screening and abortion of affected fetuses
- Congenital anomalies are the commonest cause for hospital stays over 5 days, with asthma following closely (6.2 and 6.0/1000 population, respectively)
- Cerebral palsy has an overall prevalence of 1.5–2 per 1000 live births; 9% of very-low-birthweight infants <1500 g have cerebral palsy
- Congenital blindness: 0.2/1000 live births
- Congenital sensorineural deafness: 0.8/1000 live births

Pre-school (0–4 years)

Reasons for GP consultation, England and Wales (1981–2)
Episodes per 1000 population:
Respiratory: 1188
Nervous system and sense organs: 566
Infectious disease: 447
Signs and symptoms: 390
Injuries: 124
Others: 498
Prevention: 704

- Reasons for GP consultation (5–15 years) about half the number of consultations in the same order as 0–4 years
- 9.9% of this age group have been admitted to hospital in the previous year
- 2.4% of boys and 1.8% of girls in this age band have a disability – the commonest being behaviour (13/1000), personal care (6/1000), continence (6/1000), communication (5/1000) and locomotion (5/1000)

Early school (5–9 years)

- 4.5% of boys and 3.0% of girls in this age band have a disability – the commonest being behaviour (23/1000), continence (14/1000), communication (13/1000) personal care (10/1000) and locomotion (10/1000)

Late school (10–15 years)

- 4.2% of boys and 2.9% of girls in this age band have a disability – the commonest being behaviour (25/1000), communication (13/1000), intellectual (12/1000), locomotion (11/1000) and continence (8/1000)
- 6.6% of all school children (5–15 years) have been admitted to hospital in the previous year

School leavers (16–19 years)

- The commonest disabilities in this age group are behaviour (9/1000), intellectual (9/1000), communication (8/1000), locomotion (6/1000) and continence, consciousness, personal care and hearing (4/1000 each)
- Two-thirds of children have more than one form of disability
- 8.1% of this age group have been admitted to hospital in the previous year

SPECIAL NEEDS/DISABILITY REGISTER

Every district requires two forms of information about its child population

- A child register of ALL births
    - This enables routine surveillance procedures to be carried out and monitored

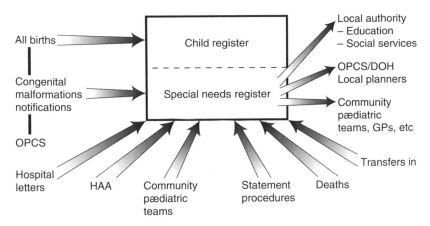

Fig. 3.1 Information sources and flow for a special-needs register.

- A special needs/disability register
  - This includes only children with clearly defined special needs which will have health and educational significance
  - It does not include children 'at risk' for such problems
  - 'Handicapped' and 'observation' registers are no longer kept by most district health authorities

Special needs/disability register

The functions of the register are:
- Monitoring/coordination of care of individual child
  - Overview of services involved
  - Monitoring changes in child's needs
  - Integral review/recall system
  - Assists liaison with involved professionals in different agencies
  - Can provide links with other information systems, e.g. social services disability registers
- Overview of services for disabled children in the district
  - Evaluation of existing services – suitability, accessibility, sufficiency
  - Identification of areas of need, e.g. communication aids in children with severe physical disability
  - Planning future services, e.g. specialist clinic for challenging behaviour in children with severe learning difficulties
- Epidemiological/research purposes
  - Surveillance of conditions
  - Monitoring trends
  - Ad hoc inquiry

Data set
- Identification of child: date of birth, address etc.
- School/nursery

- Date of entry to register
- Review date, place, person
- Diagnosis/problem – for ICD/READ coding
- Disability – category and level (mild, moderate, severe etc.) in standardized functional terms. Possible categories:
  — Mobility
  — Hand function/manipulation
  — Personal care
      Eating/drinking
      Washing/dressing
      Toileting/continence
  — Communication
  — Learning
  — Behaviour
  — Hearing
  — Vision
  — Physical health
  — Conscious state
- Named key professionals, e.g. community paediatrician, GP, educational psychologist
- Services/agencies involved
  — Health
      e.g. hospital specialists, child development centre, therapists, specialist health visitor, clinical psychology
  — Education
      e.g. special school, teacher – parent counsellor, peripatetic teachers, education welfare, statutory assessment/statement
  — Social/family
      e.g. social worker, respite care, playgroups, day nurseries, housing modification, benefits
  — Equipment
      e.g. hearing aids, wheelchair, prostheses, incontinence provision

General points
- The system must be confidential; data collected for stated purposes
- Consent of parent/carer and, where appropriate, child/young person, must be obtained for registration
- Criteria for registration must be defined, and may be:
  — Disease/diagnosis-based, i.e. all children with particular conditions are registered, e.g. all children with cerebral palsy, all children with Down's syndrome
  — Disability-based, i.e. children with certain levels of disability are registered irrespective of cause, e.g. all children with a moderate or worse level of disability in one or more categories. N.B. Several mild problems may together constitute a significant disability, and such children may warrant registration

- Register needs named person responsible for it to overview the system, answer queries, train new staff etc.
- Regular feedback to register users might be considered – this would encourage appropriate use of the system and improve data quality

SCHEME FOR THE MEDICAL ASSESSMENT OF CHILDREN WITH LEARNING DIFFICULTIES

This would provide a basis for preparing the medical contribution towards the 'statement of special educational needs' under the UK 1993 Education Act.

Checklist
- Extent and severity of learning difficulty (i.e. is it a specific disorder such as dyslexia or global delay)?
- Is it deteriorating?
- Defect of special senses?
- Language delay?
- Neurological or other chronic disorder?
- Social or behaviour concerns?

Question: Do psychologist's and teacher's reports indicate low intellectual performance?
If Yes:
- Has the child a specific syndrome associated with learning difficulties? This is suggested by positive family history and presence of dysmorphic features. The records should always contain a family tree.
  - Diagnosis may often be difficult and require expert advice from a developmental paediatrician, paediatric neurologist or clinical geneticist
  - Texts such as Smith's *Recognisable Patterns of Human Malformation,* may be helpful, as well as computer-held dysmorphology databases
  - When a syndrome has been identified, consider:
    Prognosis and natural history
    Other described associated impairments
    Genetic counselling
- Does past medical history suggest any likely causes of cerebral damage? For example:
  - Severe birth asphyxia
  - Intraventricular haemorrhage
  - Neonatal or congenital infection
  - Head injury
  - Encephalitis/meningitis
- Did parents, siblings, other relatives require special education for moderate learning difficulties?
  - Is child genetically similar?

Question: Is there any defect in the special senses?
If overlooked these can lead to an incorrect diagnosis of a learning impairment:
- Vision
    — Is visual acuity normal?
    — What is the best correction for near and distant vision?
    — Are the visual fields full?
    — What is the diagnosis?
    — Is vision likely to deteriorate?
    — Are there any genetic implications?
    — In terms of practical considerations:
      Can the child read from the blackboard?
      Can he see 'normal' size type?
      Can he see well enough to cross the road safely?
      Are there any special needs for books, lighting, low vision aids, mobility, special equipment or staffing?
      Is specialist help being received from an ophthalmologist or specialist teacher?
- Hearing
    — Is hearing normal?
    — What is the pattern of hearing loss?
    — Is it bilateral or unilateral?
    — Is it conductive or sensori-neural?
    — Does the loss fluctuate?
    — What is the diagnosis?
    — Are there genetic implications?
    — In practical terms:
      What difficulties is the child having in following lessons?
      How can the hearing be improved?
      Has the child received specialist audiological, ENT, or teaching help from special needs support teacher for the hearing impaired?
- As the child's tasks in school are principally listening and seeing, defects in these senses can greatly impair progress

Question: Is there any defect in receptive or expressive language or articulation?
Language is the vehicle for exchange of ideas.
Inner language is a necessary component of thought.
Language has an enormous social function.
Language difficulty will, therefore, cause problems in learning and behaviour.
- Ask the following questions:
    — Is English spoken at home?
    — If not, is language development normal in own tongue?
    — If English is a second language, is this poor in comparison to first?
    — Is poor language due to delay or deviant development?

— Is language delay compounded by other problems such as hearing loss, second language problems or lack of stimulation?
— In practical terms:
    Is referral to the speech therapist needed?
    Are there any related problems that require investigation?

Question: Are there any neurological problems?

- For example, epilepsy, cerebral palsy, muscular dystrophy, 'clumsy child'
    — 'Minor' problems may require careful and expert examination; major problems are unlikely to be overlooked
- Specific learning difficulties
- Is further neurological assessment required?
    — In practical terms, what are the implications in terms of:
        Mobility?
        Transport to school?
        Self-help skills?
        Medication?
        Physiotherapy/OT/speech therapy?
        Need for aids and adaptations?
        Restrictions or danger?

Question: Is there a diagnosed chronic disorder?

- For example, asthma, cystic fibrosis, diabetes, arthritis?
- How may this be influencing school progress?
    — Frequent absence from school?
        Hospital appointments
        Too ill to come
        Non-treatment absences, e.g. bad weather, 'over protection', helping mother
    — Present in school, but with poor control
        Is treatment inadequate and needing review?
        Is compliance poor?
        Review:
            Techniques of administration
            Frequency of use
            Adequacy of supplies
        Is complete control unrealistic?
        Consider additional medical, educational or social work help: e.g. help with transport, classroom assistant, home tuition, provision of new aids
    — Is treatment interfering with the level of concentration?
        e.g. some anticonvulsants and antihistamines.
        Consider changing medication if this is the case
    — Is the child adopting a 'sick role' and working below his potential level?
        If so, counselling is needed

— Are other children making unkind comments, gestures or
isolating the child?
    e.g. with regard to physical appearance, gait, use of glasses
    or aids, speech difficulties
    Management is difficult and needs to involve the whole
    class
— Is the teacher introducing unwarranted restrictions or
unnecessary differences in management – e.g. with regard to
curriculum, discipline or expectations?
— This usually means that the teacher needs much more
information and discussion
— There are frequently misconceptions, for example, children
with asthma must not do PE, and that fits are always
associated with learning difficulties

**Question: Is the social situation at home contributing towards
the child's learning difficulties?**
Social factors such as social class and legitimacy are more important
determinants of educational attainment than 'medical' factors such as
birth weight. Consider the following:

- Lack of sleep
- Hungry/inadequate diet
- Lack of appropriate past experience (stimulation)
- Physical or mental illness of the parent
- Effects of unemployment, poverty, poor housing, lack of privacy or
  space to study
- Lack of parental interest/support

These factors may be amenable to help, advice and support from the
school doctor or nurse, community or pastoral care teacher, education
welfare or social services.

**Question: Are there any emotional factors in the child and
family which are affecting performance and behaviour at school?**
Consider the effects of the following:

- General family discord, marital problems
- Young or single parent
- Truancy
- School phobia
- Depression
- Poor attention control
- Difficult temperament
- Effects of solvent abuse or other drugs
- Influence of 'video nasties' or TV
- Unrecognised effects of sexual abuse
- Presence of psychotic disorder in the child

Referral may be necessary to child psychiatrist, psychologist, social
worker or others.

Question: Are there any cultural differences in outlook, or expectations that are in conflict with attendance, attainment, or assimilation in school?
- Advice and counselling may be necessary for child, family and teachers from specialist community teachers and local community leaders

Question: Is the child bright but bored?
- These children can also do poorly in school due to boredom or excessive fear of failure
  — They may need a special curriculum

THE 1993 EDUCATION ACT (EA 1993)

Part III of the 1993 Education Act is the UK legislation dealing with special educational needs (SEN). It replaces the 1981 Education Act. Practical guidelines to all bodies involved in implementation, including health services, are contained in the Code of Practice on the Identification and Assessment of Special Educational Needs.

Principal themes of the Code of Practice:
- Any pupil who has SEN at any time must have these addressed; a continuum of needs and provision is recognised
- Greatest possible access to a broad and balanced curriculum, including the National Curriculum
- Importance of partnership between parents, children, schools, LEAs and any agencies involved
- Emphasis on earliest possible identification of SEN, including in pre-school children
- Statutory time limits on assessments
- Most children with SEN will have their needs met in mainstream, including those with statements
- Annual review of special educational provision with setting, monitoring and updating of educational targets

Definitions of special educational needs (Section 156 EA 1993)
A child has *special educational needs* if he or she has a *learning difficulty* which calls for *special educational provision* to be made for him or her.
A child has a *learning difficulty* if he or she:
- Has a significantly greater difficulty in learning than the majority of children of the same age
- Has a disability which either prevents or hinders the child from making use of educational facilities of a kind provided for children of the same age in schools within the area of the LEA
- Is under 5 and falls within the definitions above or would do so if special educational provision was not made
- A child must not be regarded as having a learning difficulty solely because the language or form of language of the home is different from the language in which he or she is or will be taught

Special educational provision means:
- For a child over 2, educational provision which is additional to, or otherwise different from, the educational provision made generally for children of the child's age in maintained schools, other than special schools, in the area
- For a child under 2, educational provision of any kind

The role of schools

All schools have responsibility for:
- Identifying children whose academic, physical, social or emotional development is giving cause for concern
- Defining areas of weakness that require extra help
- Setting and review of an individual education plan (IEP), where appropriate, designed to meet an individual child's needs, in conjunction with the parents and child
- Assessing a child's rate of progress resulting from any special educational provision
- Calling upon specialist advice from outside school where necessary
- Establishing a special needs coordinator (SENCO) for the school, whose responsibilities are:
  — Day-to-day operation of the school's SEN policy
  — Liaising with and advising fellow teachers on SEN matters
  — Coordinating school-based provision for children with SEN
  — Monitoring school's SEN register and overseeing records of all children with SEN
  — Contributing to in-service training of staff
  — Liaising with external agencies, including educational psychologists, health and social services

Assessment of SEN

Assessment is carried out using a five-stage model. Stages 1–3 are school-based. At all stages clear educational objectives are to be set, with monitoring and regular review. All details have to be recorded. Parents and child always involved.

Stages 1–3

Initial concern may be expressed by teacher, parent or other involved professionals. The teacher makes an initial assessment of SEN and consults the school's SENCO, who registers the child's SEN and decides which stage is appropriate to the child's needs. Lack of progress within a fixed timescale would result in movement to the next stage; improvement and the lessening of need for additional support would lead to the child moving to a lower stage. For children with severe problems, these early stages may be omitted.

Stage 1
- Help given in the normal classroom setting by child's own teacher – further advice and support not needed

Stage 2
- SENCO has lead responsibility for information gathering, which may include advice from outside agencies
- SENCO and teacher draw up individual education plan (IEP) to be implemented by the school
- Support from outside agencies not required

Stage 3
- SENCO has lead responsibility for information gathering which will include advice from support agencies
- SENCO, teacher and support services draw up IEP, which may actively involve outside agencies

An individual child may move between stages according to how he progresses. This will be assessed by regular reviews.

Stages 4–5
- Local Education Authority (LEA) and school share responsibility

Stage 4
- LEA consider the need for a multidisciplinary statutory assessment of SEN, and make appropriate arrangements

Stage 5
- LEA consider the need for, and if appropriate issue, a statement of SEN

Statutory assessment of SEN (Section 167 EA 1993)
LEAs have a duty to identify children in their area who may require a Statement of SEN. The Statutory Assessment of SEN is the formal process for doing this.
- LEAs may become aware of children possibly needing statutory assessment through:
  — Referral by child's school, usually through staged assessment model although immediate referral may be made in exceptional circumstances
  — Referral by another agency, e.g. Health or Social Services, particularly with pre-school children
  — Formal request from parents
- Areas that may give rise to need for assessment:
  — Learning difficulties, general or specific
  — Emotional and behavioural difficulties
  — Physical disabilities
  — Sensory impairments, hearing or vision
  — Speech and language difficulties
  — Medical conditions
- LEA requests written advice from:
  — Parents (Appendix B)
  — School (Appendix D)
  — Child Health Service (Appendix E)

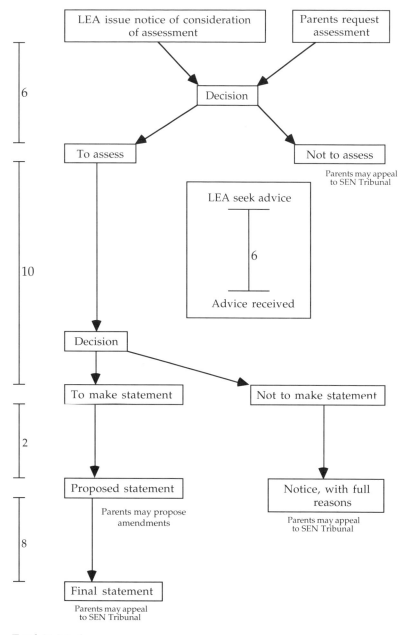

Fig. 3.2 Timescale for statutory assessment (adapted from EA 1993 Code of Practice).

    — Educational Psychology Service (Appendix F)
    — Social Services (Appendix G)
    — Any other person or agency that the LEA deem desirable (Appendix H)
- Statutory time limits exist for all parts of the assessment process (see Fig. 3.2)
- Parents have right to appeal against a decision not to assess
- Outcome of assessment:
    — Statement not issued – parents have right of appeal
    — Proposed statement issued – parents have right to make representations to LEA about content
    — Final statement issued – parents have right to appeal about content

Medical advice for statutory assessment

- Report must be returned within 6 weeks of request, unless child is unknown to the service
    — There is usually advance notification that the need for an assessment is being considered
- Must be written in easily understood language
- Should provide information on how the child's health is likely to affect his/her education
- Should be agreed in consultation with parents
- Child Health Doctor responsible for requesting and collating any necessary specialist or paramedical reports, e.g. from: speech therapy, physiotherapy, child psychiatry
- Include strengths as well as weaknesses

Content of the medical report
The following areas need to be considered, although some may not be relevant for a particular child:
- Brief description of medical problems/conditions, including relevant genetic implications
- Problem list using functional approach, e.g. mobility, hand function, communication; include positive attributes, i.e. what the child can do
- Self-help skills – toileting, feeding, dressing, washing
- Should any restrictions be placed on the child's activities?
- Include significant negatives, e.g. normality of vision or hearing
- With sensory impairments, give technical data (e.g. visual acuity, auditory thresholds) as well as functional explanation of abilities (e.g. can the child see the outline of a person, read a facial expression, hear a car coming)
- Might the child's abilities fluctuate in the short term or deteriorate in the long term?
- Summary of recommended medical facilities and resources, e.g.:
    — Medical and nursing supervision

— Physical environment, e.g. access, lighting, acoustics
— Emotional climate and social regimen
— Provision of aids, e.g. mobility, auditory, visual
— Medication
— Diet
— Health resources, e.g. speech therapy, occupational therapy, orthoptics
— Help with daily living, e.g. feeding, dressing, washing, toileting, guarding against common dangers
— Transport to school

Statement of SEN (Section 168 EA 1993)

- Main criteria for issue is when the LEA conclude that the special educational provision necessary to meet the child's need cannot reasonably be provided within the resources available to mainstream schools in the area
- Local SEN funding arrangements vary and may affect the decision to issue a statement
- Subject to annual review
  — Initiated by LEA, convened by head teacher
  — Representatives of LEA, school, parents
  — Other involved professionals may be invited
  — Written reports requested prior to meeting
  — Review report circulated after meeting

Parts of a statement:

Part 1
- Introduction
- Basic details of child and parents

Part 2
- Special educational needs
- Details of child's SEN as identified in statutory assessment

Part 3
- Special educational provision
- Objectives which the provision should meet
- Provision which the LEA consider necessary to meet the SEN specified in part 2
- Arrangements for monitoring progress of objectives

Part 4
- Placement
- Name and type of recommended school or alternative arrangements

Part 5
- Non-educational needs
- As agreed between other agencies, e.g. health

Part 6
• Non-educational provision
• Specification of agreed provision and arrangements
Appendices
• All written reports from parents, school and professionals received during the assessment process

Transitional plan
• Replaces 13+ statement review under EA 1981
• Draws together information from various people and services to plan for the young person's transition to adult life
• First annual review of a statemented child after 14th birthday (and all subsequent annual reviews) includes a transitional plan
• Arrangements, invitations and reports as for annual review, in addition:
  — Views of young person are to be obtained
  — Information from social services sought as to whether young person is disabled under the Disabled Persons Act 1986
  — Careers service representative invited

Children under 5
• DHAs and NHS Trusts must inform parents and LEA when they form the opinion that a child under 5 may have SEN. They must also inform the parents if they think a particular voluntary organization can help with their child's SEN (Section 176 EA 1993)
• LEA may expect a nursery school to follow procedures broadly similar to the school-based model
• Emphasis on liaison between health services, social services, voluntary organizations, parents and LEA
• Multidisciplinary assessment by child development centre or team may be valuable basis for assessing and discussing child's needs
• Children aged 2–5 may have a statutory assessment and may be issued with a statement using the standard procedures
• Children under 2:
  — LEA may assess if referral received from child health or social services
  — LEA must assess if parents request
  — LEA assessment need not follow statutory procedures
  — Statements will be rare

Summary of role of the community paediatrician
• To be aware of pre-school children who may have SEN and inform LEA
• General advice and support to school staff, particularly SENCOs, on health aspects of children with SEN
• Provide specific advice on stage 2 and 3 children when requested
• Provide medical advice for section 167 assessments

- Provide medical advice for annual reviews and transitional plan meetings
- Provide medical evidence for tribunal proceedings during appeals

DAY NURSERIES AND FAMILY CENTRES

- Day nurseries and family centres are often run by social services to provide day care for pre-school children
- Other forms of day care include playgroups, child-minders and educational nurseries; informal child care by the family is the commonest form
- There are approximately 35 family centre places per 1000 children under 5 in England (cf. 140 playgroup places per 1000), so that strict admission criteria apply:
  — Child at risk of abuse or neglect or suffering these
  — Severe behavioural or emotional disturbance
  — Insufficient or inadequate parental care
  — Children with moderate to severe disabilities
  — Children whose parents/carers are temporarily unable to provide care due to illness or family breakdown
- Day nursery – provides a place where under 5s are looked after for the length of working day part or full time proportional to parents' needs
- Family centre – provides more than care of child: also acts as resource for parents requiring advice, guidance and counselling; the centre may offer 'drop-in' for mothers, intensive work with children and carers separately and day care
- More day nurseries are being changed to a family centre way of working
- Both are staffed by nursery officers with NNEB qualification. They are trained in child development, child care and play. Their observations are invaluable for the community paediatrician

Role of the community paediatrician
- Awareness of problems associated with social disadvantage:-
  — Poor uptake of immunizations/child health surveillance reviews
  — Recurrent upper respiratory tract infections
  — Growth failure
  — Behaviour management difficulties (e.g. feeding, sleeping and conduct) associated with poor parenting skills or lack of social support
  — Untreated hearing loss
  — Developmental delay, particularly speech and language
  — Evidence of physical or emotional abuse
- To assess the health needs of the child and family in association with parents and nursery staff, usually as part of the assessment and review process of the nursery

- To avoid duplication of health service input by careful review of health professionals already involved with the child and family
- To plan programmes of care for the individual, including:
  — Updating of immunization
  — Behaviour-management programmes
  — Advice about nutrition and growth
  — Coordination of services for children with disability – family centres are increasingly developing facilities for multi-disciplinary review meetings
- Teaching and support of nursery staff, e.g. recognition of signs of child abuse, growth measurement technique
- Help develop guidelines:
  — Infectious disease policy
    Diarrhoea, especially rotavirus, is very common
    Handwashing facilities must be inspected and staff made aware of appropriate hygiene measures
    Closure of nursery should be avoided where possible
  — Medicines in nursery policy
    Nurseries may have different guidelines for the issue of medicines to children
    Private and local authority nurseries often differ
    Important that staff are supported in giving medicines, e.g. antibiotics, anticpileptics and inhalers
    Children are placed at an additional disadvantage if medicines are not administered

Guidance for doctors working in nurseries and family centres
- A flexible approach is necessary
  — Meeting with parents during a 'drop-in' session
  — Observing a child, whom nursery staff are worried about, during play
  — Arranging to see siblings at the nursery to save different members of the family being seen at more than one consultation
  — Try to avoid dwelling solely on the pathological. Parents are often distrustful of authority and therefore you need to be positive where possible about parenting abilities and their child's achievements
  — Attendance at case reviews and case conferences is very useful and helps to build up relationships
  — Nursery nurses are excellent observers and their knowledge of normal child development may be better than yours – ask for their support!

EDUCATION FOR CHILDREN WITH SPECIAL NEEDS

Funding
- Headteachers manage their own school's budget under Local Management for Schools (LMS) and decide how money is spent

- Basic funding depends on number of pupils attending the school
- Extra funds for special needs allocated on an individual school basis; usually depends on number of children receiving free school meals
- Additional funds may be available for schools in areas of deprivation
- Further funding available for an individual child with identified special educational needs; this is usually done though a statement of special educational needs
- There is local variation in funding arrangements

The National Curriculum
- Applies to all pupils of compulsory school age in all maintained schools, including grant-maintained mainstream and special schools
- Organized on the basis of four key stages (Education Reform Act 1988, amended by Education Act 1993):

	Pupils' ages	*Year groups*
Key Stage 1	5–7	1–2
Key Stage 2	7–11	3–6
Key Stage 3	11–14	7–9
Key Stage 4	14–16	10–11

The following subjects are included in England:
Key Stages 1 and 2
English, maths, science, technology (design and technology, and information technology), history, geography, art, music, physical education
Key Stage 3
As above, plus a modern foreign language
Key Stage 4
English, maths, science, physical education, technology (design and technology, and information technology), modern foreign language

For each key stage and subject
Programmes of study set out what pupils should be taught
Attainment targets set out expected standards of performance

Assessment at key stages 1–3
- All subjects except art, music, PE
    — National tests carried out at the end of each key stage – standard assessment tasks (SATs)
    — Eight-level descriptions (grades) of increasing difficulty
    — Levels give indication of performance in relation to average expected for age, e.g.:
        level 2 targets will be average for key stage 1 SATs (7 years)
        level 4 targets will be average for key stage 2 SATs (11 years)
        level 5 and 6 targets will be average for key stage 3 SATs (14 years)
    — Additional level above level 8 for exceptional performance
- Art, music, PE

— *End of key stage descriptions* set out standard performance expected of all pupils at end of each key stage
— Description of exceptional performance provided for art and music at the end of key stage 3 and in PE at the end of key stage 4

Assessment at key stage 4 is mainly by public examination, e.g. GCSE

Special educational needs
• Should be provided for within the broad framework of the national curriculum
• Appropriately challenging work should be provided at each key stage
• Sections of the national curriculum may be modified or disapplied if necessary, either temporarily by the head teacher's direction or through a statement of special educational needs

Children with special educational needs in different types of school

In ordinary mainstream school:
• Most children with special needs can be educated within the mainstream school system
  — For example, most children with epilepsy, heart disorders, diabetes, asthma, cystic fibrosis, bleeding disorders are at mainstream school
• Medical information and guidance to individual teachers from the school doctor and nurse is needed. Many specialist hospital clinics have liaison nurses who will visit schools to discuss particular issues, e.g. diabetic liaison nurses
• Some children with more disabling conditions can be educated in mainstream school if adequate ancillary help is provided, e.g.:
  — Classroom special needs support assistant
  — Physiotherapy/occupational therapy advice/support
  — School nurse on campus
  — Help from special advisory teacher, such as teacher of the deaf or visually impaired
  — Outreach support – teachers from local special schools giving advice to school staff or working with child
• Structural alterations may need to be considered, e.g. ramps, rails, suitable toilet facilities; these must be planned well in advance of school entry
• Specialist equipment/aids may be required, e.g. mobility aids, catheterization equipment
• Need to ensure appropriate provision for child at dinner time and breaks, not just during lessons
• May require transport to and from school
• There is a tendency for more children with special needs of all kinds, but particularly learning difficulties, to be educated in mainstream schools. Families and teaching staff need support and advice regarding appropriate provision and resourcing

In special units (individual needs centres) attached to ordinary mainstream schools:
- These usually cater for a specific disability
- Unit has specially trained staff and appropriate equipment
- Children spend most of the time in ordinary classes
- Children can be withdrawn for special tuition, and can receive additional specialist help with mobility, incontinence, communication, etc.
- Examples:
  — Unit for hearing impaired with amplification and other communication aids
  — Unit for visual handicap with special aids resources
  — Unit for the physically handicapped constructed on one level or with adaptations for mobility and with the help of a school nurse and physiotherapist
- Units cater for small numbers of children
- School premises adapted to children's needs
- Mainstream staff have ready access to specialist advice regarding the special-needs children
- Prevent social isolation and give access to broad curriculum as well as special resources
- Children regarded as being in mainstream education and not in special school

In special day school:
- Serve a defined catchment area and usually specialize in a specific area of need
- Children with similar types of special needs can be educated together
- Examples:
  — Physical handicap
  — Learning difficulty – moderate or severe
  — Difficult behaviour
- Transport to school is provided
- School premises adapted to children's needs
- Schools have small classes and specialized teaching staff and other resources
- The more severely disabled children usually attend these schools, where education in mainstream is not possible
- Schools usually have attached therapists and nurses

In special residential school:
- These schools exist for a variety of reasons:
  — In rural areas where a long distance has to be travelled to reach an appropriate school
  — To provide specialist education for relatively rare disabilities, e.g. severe visual impairment
  — To provide education for children whose physical or other

handicap is so severe as to make management at home
difficult or impossible
— Where home circumstances are such that a child's
educational progress is adversely affected by remaining at
home
- Some special schools combine day and residential facilities

In other units:
- Attached to hospitals:
  - Ordinary children's wards
  - Long-stay, e.g. orthopaedic
  - Child and adolescent psychiatric units
- Tutorial classes for children with difficulties coping emotionally in
ordinary school (also sanctuary classes)
- Assessment units
  - For entrants where there is considerable doubt about the
nature of their special educational needs
  - A period of observation and assessment in an educational
setting will enable an appropriate recommendation to be made
  - Units may be attached to ordinary or special school
  - Children may be admitted 'without prejudice' or may already
be the subject of a statement
- Pupil referral units (PRUs) for children with emotional and
behaviour problems or discipline problems, who are unable to
integrate into a normal school structure and organization and for
whom a small, free-standing unit might be appropriate
- Units for pregnant schoolgirls

At home:
- Home tuition may be provided:
  - During recovery from illness or injury
  - Emotional problems
  - Pregnancy
  - Terminal illness

Mainstream versus special schools
Special schools
- Small classes
- Child's achievements appropriate to range of that of peers
- Specialized teaching at hand
- Concentration of appropriate resources
- Adequate nursing and therapy support
- Are segregated from normal peer group
- May be overprotective
- Parents can share experiences

Mainstream schools
- Larger classes
- Specialized remedial teaching less accessible

- Often less support from therapists and nurses
- Greater variety of courses
- Greater stimulation from peer competition
- Identification as neighbourhood school
- May be overprotective of disabled child
- Child can become isolated within the school
- May be over-tolerant of deviant behaviour
- Staff may have no previous experience of teaching special needs children
- Special needs services may be under-resourced
- Other children have experience of peers with disability
- Teachers may have less time for other children

Special needs in mainstream – summary of the role of the school doctor
- Be aware of pre-school children who are likely to have special educational needs in good time for appropriate provision to be made
- Provide advice to school staff on medical aspects of child's special needs; disclosure of medical information to teachers, and their need to know, must be discussed with parents
    — Diagnoses
    — Practical implications
    — Likely progress of condition
    — Treatment needed
    — Health follow-up required
- Regular liaison with school's special educational needs coordinator (SENCO)
- Provide medical advice for statutory assessments and transitional plans
- Assist liaison between school and other involved health professionals, e.g. hospital specialists, therapists
- Provide ongoing support to child, family and teaching staff; continuity in this role is important
- Advice to careers service and Disabled Persons Act services
- Be involved in multidisciplinary case reviews at school, including statutory reviews, which may involve:
    — Ensuring that all relevant health professionals are invited, as well as education, social services, voluntary sector, parents/carers and, where appropriate, child or young person
    — Ensuring that all aspects of the national curriculum are addressed, including PE
    — Ensuring that the child is allowed to take part in normal non-teaching activities, e.g. dinner times, break times, trips
    — Planning moves from infants to junior, and from junior to secondary
    — Particular issues to consider may include:
        Social integration in school

Child's emotional needs, including self-esteem, feelings of
achievement or failure
Independence skills
Mobility
Seating
Carrying books etc.
Access to all of school
Any structural alterations required
Aids and appliances
Hand function
Communication
Toileting
Changing
Meals
Medication
Tiredness
Transport to and from school
Leisure
Welfare rights and benefits

THE SCHOOL DOCTOR TO THE SPECIAL SCHOOL

Every school for children with special needs should have a doctor who
visits regularly. This doctor may be the 'lead paediatrician' responsible
for all aspects of management or will need to liaise closely with that
person. Children with complex needs may have several consultants, for
example paediatrician, neurosurgeon, urologist, orthopaedic surgeon,
neurologist, ENT surgeon, ophthalmologist. Additionally, many others
are frequently key figures in assessment and daily management;
examples are physiotherapy, occupational therapy, speech therapy,
clinical psychology, dietetics.

The framework of this doctor's work is:
• To see children before they start school in order to get to know
  them and their families
  — To discuss the implications of the child's medical condition
    with teachers, therapists and nurses
  — To establish a link between the school and other
    paediatricians looking after the child for example to share
    information or to make arrangements for emergency
    admission from school if this is needed

• To see each child annually to:
  — Review medical problems affecting education, vision, hearing,
    epilepsy and its treatment
  — Review mobility with physiotherapists

— Review sensory problems
— Discuss with parents any problems arising in the home:
   Mobility
   Independence
   Nursing
   Behaviour
   Sexual problems
— To review diagnosis in doubtful cases
- To undertake day-to-day medical management through either school, community, where that doctor has a lead role or in conjunction with that person
- To give support and advice to parents and staff
- To provide advice to the careers service or social services department on school leaving about:
   — Effect of medical condition on suitability for employment
   — Need for medical care after school leaving
   — This should be in a suitable form to be given also to the young person or his family
- To provide day-to-day medical management of the child at school and to give support and advice to staff and parents

Transitional care plan

- This aims:
   — To make plans for the next stage of the young person's development by reviewing:
      Diagnosis – possible genetic advice
      Sensory and motor problems
      Aids to mobility and adaptations to the home
      Any medical treatment
- Theoretically provides a smooth transition from school to adulthood services and should be done when the child is aged 13–14 years; this involves education, social services and the family, with health professionals providing relevant contributions

Doctor's role with the:

Young person
- As annual review AND in addition
- How can they contribute towards their own transition plan and make positive decisions for the future, including hopes/aspirations?
- What information do they need to make informed choices?

Family
- What are the parental expectations?
- How can they contribute towards the aspirations above?
- Do they require practical help in terms of aids, etc?
- Inform them of new allowances available in adulthood which may need to be claimed in advance of the person reaching 16 to avoid payment delay

Education
- The headteacher to provide a list of students at the start of each academic year together with possible dates for multi-disciplinary meetings; this may need to be negotiated locally depending on teachers workloads, but will aid the planning of your assessments
- The headteacher should coordinate the overall care plan after you have provided the medical component

Social services
- The Disability Implementation Act should aid the transition and some areas have teams which deal specifically with this. Check if your area has a contact name/team
- Be aware of allowances available to 16 year olds
- Obtain consent for a copy of your educational statement to be sent to social services
- Social services are invited to the transitional care meetings

Other health professionals
- Obtain and coordinate reports as in 'educational statement'
- Reports should be available to the parents and hence understandable without jargon

Suggested training activity
- Visit colleges of further education and speak to respective special educational needs coordinator. Particularly useful when discussing transitional care plan in terms of training environment for disabled teenagers, accommodation and local schemes to help achieve independence
- Meet careers guidance officer and local social service contact who can arrange/advise on allowances/respite/clubs for disabled adults
- Meet associated health professionals, i.e. school physiotherapist/OT/speech therapist and also adult-associated specialists if available, i.e. occupational psychologists, rehabilitation medicine specialist and adult physician/psychiatrist responsible for maintaining care into adulthood

LEARNING DISABILITY

Chief causes in children
- Chromosomal abnormalities
    - Down's syndrome
    - Other trisomies
    - Deletions
    - Fragile X
- Single gene abnormalities
    - Biochemical defects, e.g. PKU
    - Tuberose sclerosis
    - Other dysmorphic syndromes

- Perinatal infections
  - Rubella
  - Toxoplasmosis
  - Cytomegalovirus
  - Herpes
  - Neonatal meningitis
- Postnatal infections
  - Meningitis
  - Encephalitis
  - Severe infections in young babies
- Dysmorphic syndromes
  - Known syndromes
  - Known associations
  - Unknown associations
- Perinatal problems
  - Hypoxia
  - IVH
  - Convulsions
- Injury
  - Accidental
  - Non-accidental
- Unknown origin
  - 20–30% in most series

Early intervention
- Parent counselling
  - To come to terms with handicap
  - To participate in therapy and teaching
  - To foresee and prevent problems in behaviour
- To treat or minimize treatable causes, e.g. hearing/visual problems
- Nursery education appropriate to needs
  - To benefit from early childhood education, meet peer group and learn to share

Referral to education authority to consider child's special needs and to provide pre-school teaching advice
Medical advice for statement of educational needs should include:
- Mobility
  - As for physical disability, but motivational factors also need to be addressed
- Hand function
  - As for physical disability
- Continence
- Whether condition is progressive
- Any pre-dispositions, e.g. hearing loss in Down's children
- Epilepsy (often hard to control in severely multiply handicapped children)
- Transport to and from school

- Need for aids
  - Seating
  - Feeding
  - Communication
- Need for therapy

Annual review
- As for physical disability
- Health promotion needs should not be forgotten (including sex education)
- Recreational needs are equally important and should also be specifically addressed
- Transitional plan at first annual review after 14th birthday: see Education Act 1993

Review on leaving school
- Family and young person's understanding of medical condition
- Advice to social services (Disabled Persons Act team), careers or further education departments
- Benefits
- Transfer of medical care to adult or young adult services
- A written summary is very useful at this stage, with copies for the family and GP
- If there are genetic implications that have not been considered at the time of the transitional plan, this presents a further opportunity for counselling to be made available to the young person and family

PHYSICAL DISABILITY

Main causes in children
- Cerebral palsy
- Spina bifida (decreasing numbers)
- Duchenne muscular dystrophy
- Other degenerative neuromuscular conditions

Early intervention
- Early education
- Groups to overcome isolation
- Voluntary agencies
- Lack of mobility restricts learning; therefore, aids to mobility may help developmental progress
- Therapy to increase mobility and teach daily living skills

Referral to education authority to consider child's special needs
Medical evidence for statement of educational needs should consider:
- Mobility
  - Does child need wheelchair, calipers, crutches?
  - Does he/she walk with difficulty?
  - Can he/she manage stairs? If so, how easily and how fast?

- Hand function
  - Is this normal/clumsy?
  - Can child hold pencil, knife, fork?
  - One-sided weakness produces problems with writing, dressing, toileting
- Continence
  - Can child use toilet independently/with adult help?
  - Does he/she require any form of incontinence appliance?
- Need for therapy
- Need for nursing help – medication
- Epilepsy
  - Frequency and type of fit
  - Medication
- Transport to and from school
- Need for aids
  - Seating
  - Special cutlery
  - Communication aids
- Any sensory problems?
- Whether condition is progressive

Annual review of children with physical disabilities
This is undertaken with parent, school nurse and therapist in full cooperation with teaching staff:
- Medical
  - Intercurrent illness
  - Progression of signs and symptoms
- Educational
  - Progress in school related to medical condition
- Aids
  - Adaptations which might be needed as the child grows
- Social considerations

Transitional care plan (see School Doctor to the Special School)
- Review diagnosis – especially with regard to genetic counselling of young person and family
- Look forward to further independence training in preparation for leaving school

Review on school leaving
- Young person's understanding of his/her condition
- Advice to careers or further education department
- Advice and certification re allowances
- Transfer of medical care to adult services

HEARING SCREENING AND TESTING

- Incidence of significant bilateral sensorineural hearing loss 1–2 per thousand births

- 25% pre-school children have one or more episodes of otitis media with effusion (OME)

Neonate
- Some forms of congenital deafness may progress after birth and not be detectable in the neonatal period, e.g. congenital rubella, CMV, some types of genetically determined sensorineural hearing loss

Methods
- Auditory response cradle (ARC) – computer-assisted assessment of infant response to sound (e.g. movements, change in respirations)
- Auditory brainstem responses (ABR) – recording and analysis of EEG signals evoked in response to sound
- Oto-acoustic emissions (OAE) – the auditory echo emitted by a normal cochlear

Screening may be:
- Universal
- Selective for high-risk babies, e.g. low birth weight, severe asphyxia, family history of deafness, cranio-facial abnormality, congenital infection

District policies vary

Birth to 1 year
Clues list for hearing:
- Sheet given to parents at birth visit (see Fig. 3.3)
- Advises parents what to look for at different ages
- Very effective if parental concerns acted upon by prompt referral to the children's hearing assessment centre

6–7 months

Distraction test
- Until recently, this test was universal. The value of this test as a screening procedure is being questioned and some Districts have abandoned it on the basis of low sensitivity and high numbers of false positives; they suggest an enquiry about parental concern with an audiological assessment of those with impaired language development, a history of middle-ear disease or developmental or behaviour problems. If neonatal screening is universal, it may be easier to adopt a selective test at this time; if it is not, then investment is needed in staff training and audit of the results of this procedure. The key points seem to be eliciting and responding to parental suspicions and a well organized and assessible district audiological service

Test requires
- Trained staff
- Quiet environment
- Absence of other clues, e.g. perfume, shadows, creaking floor – deaf children are very alert to clues
- Test can be used up to 18 months of age

CAN YOUR BABY HEAR YOU?

Here is a checklist of some of the signs you can look for in your baby's first year:-

Tick if
Response
Present

Shortly after birth

Your baby should be startled by a sudden loud noise and he should blink or open his eyes widely to such sounds.

☐

By 1 Month

He should show the additional response of becoming still if you make a sudden prolonged sound.

☐

By 3 Months

He should quieten or smile to the sound of your voice even when he cannot see you. He may also turn his head or eyes towards you if you come up from behind and speak to him from the side.

☐

By 6 Months

He should turn immediately to your voice across the room or to very quiet noises made on each side.

☐

By 9 Months

He should listen attentively to familiar everyday sounds and search for very quiet sounds made out of sight. He should also show pleasure in babbling loudly and tunefully.

☐

By 12 Months

He should show some response to his own name and to other familiar words. He may also respond to 'no' and 'bye bye'.

☐

IF YOU SUSPECT THAT YOUR BABY IS NOT HEARING NORMALLY EITHER BECAUSE YOU CANNOT PLACE A DEFINITE TICK AGAINST THE ITEMS ABOVE OR FOR SOME OTHER REASON THEN CONTACT YOUR HEALTH VISITOR FOR ADVICE. SHE WILL PERFORM A SIMPLE HEARING SCREENING TEST ON YOUR BABY BETWEEN SEVEN AND NINE MONTHS OF AGE AND WILL BE ABLE TO HELP AND ADVISE YOU AT ANY TIME IF YOU ARE CONCERNED ABOUT YOUR BABY AND HIS DEVELOPMENT.

Fig. 3.3 Hints for parents produced by Dr Barry McCormick, Nottingham Hearing Services Centre.

Sounds:
- High frequency
    - — 'Manchester' rattle
    - — Consonant 's' sound
    - — Electronic warbler at 4000 Hz
- Low frequency
    - — Voice without consonants, 'oo' or hum
    - — Electronic warbler at 500 Hz
- Minimal levels
    - — <35 db at 1 m
    - — Check with sound level meter

Results:
- 1st fail – retest within 1 month at latest, or refer if concerns
- 2nd fail – refer to children's hearing assessment centre

A new automated version of the test, which requires only one person has been developed.

5–6 years

Pure tone audiometry
- All children should be tested in school
- 'Sweep test' requires response at 30 db at 500 Hz, 1 kHz, 2 kHz, 4 kHz
- If fail at any frequency, full audiogram is performed and referred to the doctor

Hearing testing at other times

- In addition to the screening programme certain groups should be tested:
  - Recurrent middle-ear disease
  - Language concerns
  - Post-meningitis
  - Parental concerns
- Hearing testing in pre-school children is difficult and should be carried out only by trained professionals, preferably those who are doing it regularly
- The following tests may be used for particular age groups:

18–30 months

Cooperative testing
- 'Where are your shoes?'
- 'Give this to Mummy'
- 'Give it to dolly'
- 'Give it to teddy'
- Test requires
  - Minimal levels <40 db at 1 m – check with sound level meter
  - Careful exclusion of visual clues
- Difficult age to test as a routine
- Distraction test still needed for children with developmental delay

2.5–5 years

Auditory discrimination test
- For example, McCormick toy discrimination test, picture cards (Stycar or RNID)
- Tests discrimination between similar sounding words
- Test requires response at <40 db at 1 m either side – check with sound level meter
- Child must not be able to lip read from tester
- Clues such as looking at the object requested or asking for the objects on a picture card in a fixed sequence must be avoided

Performance test
- Child is taught to respond in a particular way to hearing a sound, e.g. put 'men' in a boat, bricks in a box (the activity must be a quiet one)
- Sounds may be 'go', 'ss', warble tone or pure tones
- Child must respond <40 db at 1 m either side – check with sound level meter
- Needs variable interval between test sounds as fixed interval will give many clues

Audiometry
- Standard pure-tone audiogram with headphones
- If child is sufficiently mature and cooperative

HEARING PROBLEMS

Hearing problems fall into two categories:
- Conductive
    - Up to 60 db loss
    - Often low tone> high tone loss
    - Usually due to middle-ear effusion
- Sensorineural
    - Any degree of loss
    - Generally flat loss or high tone
    - Many causes, often genetically determined

Infants

Suspect hearing loss if:
- Parents suspect loss
- Child fails health visitor's testing
- Major neonatal problems
- Post-meningitis
- Deafness in immediate family
- Loss of babbling
- Recurrent ear infections
- Associated problems, e.g. craniofacial abnormalities
- Young children with suspected moderate or severe losses should be referred to the children's hearing assessment centre as soon as possible
- N.B. Normal babble can occur in profoundly deaf children

Older children

Suspect hearing loss if:
- Parents suspect loss
- They fail screening tests at school
- They have recurrent ear infections
- Speech is poor
- Educational progress is poor

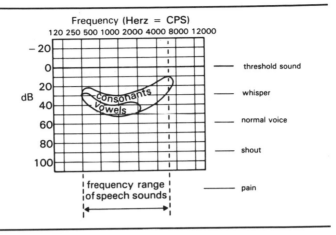

Fig. 3.4 Measurement of deafness.

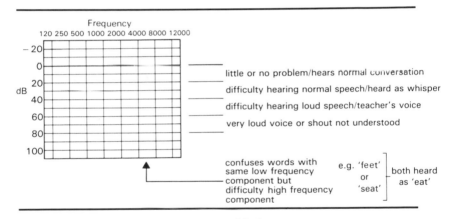

Fig. 3.5 Disability associated with various degrees of deafness.

- Behaviour problems
- Associated problems, e.g. cleft palate, Down's syndrome

For mild loss (25–35 db):

- Is it intermittent or recent in onset?
- Is speech, behaviour, school progress satisfactory?
- If yes: inform school, advise parents, follow up
- If no: consider intervention – if there is otitis media with effusion (OME), 25–50% will improve spontaneously
  - If spontaneous resolution does not occur and hearing impairment is giving rise to disability, co-trimoxazole for 4 weeks can be effective

— Surgical referral necessary if hearing loss becomes moderate or severe, persistent and symptomatic, i.e problems with learning, behaviour or language

For moderate loss (40–60 db)
- Assess as above, but likely to need referral to ENT department unless clearly temporary, e.g. acute otitis media

For severe loss (>60 db)
- Bilateral
    — Refer urgently to children's hearing assessment centre
    — Consider false positives due to poor performance of the test if clinical picture does not match audiogram; expert assessment still required
    — Unilateral, refer to ENT department
- The audiogram is only one factor in assessing the child; treat the child not the audiogram
- The school must be informed of all children with moderate and severe losses, and any children with mild losses who have learning or other difficulties
- Hearing losses may cause dangers when crossing the road
- If the child is having speech therapy, let the therapist know the level of loss
- If the loss in a pre-school child is likely to give rise to special education needs, make sure that the educational psychologist knows about the child

MANAGEMENT OF THE DEAF CHILD

Team approach: family+
- Audiologist
- ENT surgeon
- Teacher of the deaf
- Speech therapist
- Educational psychologist
- Social worker
- Paediatrician/neurologist
- Ophthalmologist
- Geneticist (50% of severe deafness inherited)

Assessment includes:
- Degree of hearing loss
- Cause of deafness
- Consequences of deafness (for child, family and school)
- General paediatric assessment
    — Syndrome?
    — Associated conditions?
    — Is vision normal?

— Is development normal?
— Any other problems?
— Personality of child
- Language development
- Educational attainment
- Social assessment
  — Strengths and weaknesses
  — Supports
  — Home conditions
  — Family composition

Management includes:
- Parent counselling and support
- Early oral training
- Provision of aids
- Medical and surgical management of conductive problems
- Appropriate educational provision
- Genetic counselling

ADVICE FOR TEACHERS OF CHILDREN WITH MILD/MODERATE HEARING LOSSES

- The child should sit near the front of the class
- If there is deafness in only one ear, the better ear should face the teacher
- The child will be helped if he can see the teacher's face
- The child should be allowed to turn around to see the faces of other children participating in class discussions
- It is not necessary for the teacher to shout or use exaggerated lip movements
- The child should be encouraged to take part in all activities
- In games, the child may miss some instructions
- There are hazards crossing the road – the child must look for oncoming traffic
- The child may be aware of a quiet voice, but miss the clarity of speech:
  — Some words may be missed altogether
  — Other words may be confused, e.g. 'choose' and 'shoes'
- The hearing loss is likely to fluctuate from day to day
  — On good days it may appear to be normal
  — On bad days there is considerable difficulty
- The problem will be greater in noisy surroundings
- The problem will be greater if more than one person is speaking at a time
- If one ear is affected more than the other, the child may have difficulty in locating sounds and in understanding speech from the poor side

- The teacher should be aware of the increased concentration required by the child to follow speech
- Any special attention should be handled as unobtrusively as possible
- Patience is required if the child repeatedly misunderstands
- If the child has a hearing aid the teacher needs to know how to check that it is switched on!

LANGUAGE

- Language development is a reliable indicator of future educational progress
- Language is the most complex of human skills and is necessary for thought as well as communication
- Language problems frequently lead to behaviour problems
- Problems can exist in the following areas:
  - Concentration
    How distractable is the child?
    Is attention poor all the time or can the child be encouraged to concentrate by firm handling?
    How does the child respond one-to-one compared to in a group?
  - Symbolic understanding (inner language)
    1 year – demonstrates use of life-size object, e.g. cup, spoon
    15 months – demonstrates use of miniature objects
    18 months – relates two objects, e.g. gives doll a drink
    30 months – acts out with miniature toys
  - Articulation
    - Functional difficulties in production of speech sounds
    - Most common and least serious problem
  - Expression
    - Defect in use of spoken language
    - Defect in use of speech sounds
  - Comprehension
    Least common and most serious
  - Social use of language, e.g. autistic spectrum disorders
  - Rhythm, e.g. stammer
  - Voice, e.g. hoarseness
  - Or any combination of the above
- Incidence of language problems at school entry (age 5)
    5% – unintelligible
    1% – delayed development
    0.1% – severe (deviant) language disorder
    0.01% – comprehension disorder

Causes of speech and language problems
- Developmental delay
  - Speech and language delay, with or without delayed social skills

— Generalized developmental delay
— Language delay is often the first problem to be identified in children who go on to have learning difficulties
- Hearing problem
  — High tone loss and intermittent loss due to otitis media with effusion (OME), can be missed – both can lead to speech problems
  — OME can cause delay
  — High tone loss can cause omission of consonant sounds or confusion, e.g. 'choose' and 'shoes'
- Environment
  — Lack of language stimulation – common and amenable to intervention
  — Children of deaf parents and those from bilingual families usually have normal language development, but will have more problems if there are other difficulties
- Structural
  — Cleft palate, nasal obstruction, palato-pharyngeal incompetence, malocclusion of the jaws, hypoplasia of the tongue, macroglossia
- Neurological
  — Cerebral palsy
  — Muscular defects, e.g. myotonic dystrophy, myasthenia gravis
- Psychiatric
  — Elective mutism, autism
- Specific language disorders
  — Boys > girls
  — Often a family history
  — May be clumsy and have reading and writing problems

Assessment

History
- Family history of language problems
- Social history
- Birth history
- PMH of otitis media, meningitis, encephalitis
- Feeding problems
- General and language development
- Opportunities for language use, e.g. stories, picture books, play, everyday use of language
- Specific details from parents:
  — When and how much parents talk to the child and *listen and respond to what he says*, i.e. how do they reinforce use of language?
  — How does the child get what he wants, e.g. gesture, helps himself, takes parent's hand to object, language?
  — Is he frustrated by lack of language?

— Is English the language used in the home? If not, what is?
— If family do not speak English at home, are there any problems in his own language?
— What language is used in everyday life by the child – vocabulary, word combinations, intelligibility, jargon?
— At what age did these stages in language development take place?
— What simple verbal commands from parents can the child usually follow?
— Do the parents suspect any hearing loss?
— Does he talk to himself during play?
— Presence or absence of symbolic play

Examination
• Observe level of language interaction between parent and child
• Does the child use non-verbal clues to aid comprehension – lip reading, gesture, voice inflection, situational?
• Observe the child's social interaction – eye contact, facial expressions, empathy, turn taking, social timing
• Is there any impairment in attention?
• Observe the child's behaviour – distractibility, hyperactivity, mannerisms, obsessions, pre-occupations, ritualistic behaviour; does he look for adult's responses to his actions?
• General development – is language development in line with other abilities?
• Examination with particular reference to movements of the lips, tongue, palate, and occlusion of teeth
    — Nasal obstruction – difficulty with 'n', 'm', 'ng', no air entry when asked to sniff; adenoidal enlargement; displacement of nasal septum; chronic rhinitis
    — Cleft palate or sub-mucous cleft – nasal escape of air when utters 'e' sound (clouds mirror or moves cotton wool)
    — Malocclusion of jaws – difficulties with 's' and 's'-blends; micrognathia – small lower jaw; prognathism – protrusion of lower jaw
    — Tongue – congenital hypoplasia (small immobile tongue); macroglossia, e.g. in Down's syndrome, Hurler's syndrome, Beckwith syndrome
    — Neurological
        50% of children with cerebral palsy have articulation problems
        Look for spasticity giving rise to slow laborious speech
        Look for involuntary movements
        Look for feeding problems, drooling
• Assess hearing

Clinical assessment of language
See Table 3.1 for details of expected language development.

• Comprehension
    — Identifies objects on request – 'give me the doll, cup, spoon'

— Links objects and ideas – 'put the doll on the chair'
— Understands more complicated concepts: 'show me the biggest balloon'
- Expression
  — Names simple objects or pictures
  — Length of word combinations
  — Use of nouns, verbs, adjectives, adverbs
  — Echolalia (repetition of words heard) – should not persist beyond 30 months
  — Note examples of sentence structure – normal, delayed or deviant
  — Note omission of parts of words (may indicate hearing problems)
  — Note substitution of consonants, e.g. 'too' for 'shoe'. Substitution of similar sounds reflects immaturity, substitution of dissimilar sounds is deviant
  — Note quality of voice, e.g. hoarse, nasal
  — Note presence of stutter (intervention not recommended below 8 years of age)
  — Some sounds are commonly not correct at age 5 – 'sh', 'cl', 'ds', 's', 'ch', 'sm', 'sp', 'str', 'sh', 'th', difficulties with these are not an abnormality
- Referral
  — Speech therapists like to see children early
  — Refer for speech therapy assessment as soon as it is clear there is a problem
  — All children with no single words by 2 years or no two-word sentences by 3 years should have been referred
  — If poor environment is thought to be a cause, consider use of toy library, simple home programme or day care

Autism
- There is a spectrum of autistic disorder with a varying range of severity
- Assessment probably best carried out using a multidisciplinary approach involving professionals with experience of autism, eg developmental paediatrician, psychiatrist, psychologist, speech therapist
- The following three features are necessary for the diagnosis, all present by 30 to 36 months:
  — *Global impairment of language*, involving failure to code in any of the early communicative modes:
    Facial expression
    Gesture and other body language
    Spoken language
    Social timing, i.e. mechanism required for use of these languages in flow of dialogue (i.e. for conversation)
  — *Impairment of social relationships*, in particular a failure of social empathy; includes:

Unwillingness to share social gaze (eye contact)
Unwillingness to be touched
Failure to comment on or show things to others (either
verbally or pre-verbally)
(Later) failure to respond when addressed as a member of a
group
— *Evidence of rigidity of thought processes*, including linguistic
thought:
Resistance to change (though not to novelty) – includes
difficulty in adapting concepts to include new information
Obsessions and pre-occupations, including obsessions with
certain patterns (e.g. spirals, converging lines) to the
exclusion of meaning
Ritualistic behaviour
Echolalia, and thence pronoun reversal
Stereotypic activities replace play
Clumsiness, poor imitation of action patterns
Poor incidental learning
Minimal symbolic play (pretending)

Age	Comprehension	Expressive language	Phonology
1;0	Situational understanding. Looks appropriately at familiar named object/person. Understands a few object labels.	Tuneful babbling. Simple intonation patterns. Recognisable single words beginning.	Several different sounds in babble.
1;6	Understands several everyday object labels, e.g. chair, baby, man.	Mainly single word utterances, e.g. milk, mama, want, go, more, why; (two word utterances beginning). Specific vocalisations to obtain needs, express emotions.	
2;0	Understands many single words. Increasing receptive vocabulary. Early two-word comprehension, e.g. *'daddy's hat'*, 'put the *spoon* on the *table'*.	Two element utterances amongst many single words. Some simple three word utterances beginning; e.g. want red shirt; mummy sit chair.	p b m n w
2;6	Understands most two word commands, e.g. *wash dolly* (action + object); *dirty shoe* (attribute + object); *walk door* (action + place); *teddy sleep* (person + action).	Many two word and some three word utterances. Verbs, adjectives, pronouns appearing; e.g. in your cup baby is crying my little teddy	t d k g ng h
3;0	Understands: three-word commands; e.g. *throw ball daddy* *wash dolly's face*; some simple prepositions (in, under); big/little; maybe; some simple colours.	2–4 element utterances (may be more than four words). Shows prepositions, articles and pronouns; e.g. Daddy's kicking the ball now; Me go in kitchen in a minute.	f s l y
3;6	Four word comprehension; e.g. *wash doll's hair bathroom* *spoon under little cup* in/on/under. boy/girl/man. Maybe colours (incl. black and white).	Formation of complex sentences with many words, e.g. because, and, but (may be some omission of grammatical words; pronouns may be immature).	
4;0	Wide range of four word comprehension involving colours, prepositions, size, verbs, etc. Understands wh- words, comparatives, related sentences, e.g. wash the table and wash the chair; wash the cups and put them in the cupboard.	Eradication of immature forms.	sh v z r ch j sp st sc etc. pl br etc.
4;6	Comprehension of *tense* — present, past; pronouns, long/short etc; can't.	Completion of syntax stylistic variations emerging; e.g. it's green, you see, there are cows in the field. I've got a new dress, anyway.	gr fr
5;0	Comprehension of embedded phrase, e.g. the boy with no hat is digging. Harder prepositions — between, in front. Singular/plural.		th (maybe) str fl

Notes: The tables should be used with caution. These age-norms should be accurate within a ± six month range from the age stated. Where a child is obviously well below the expectations for his age, it would be wise to ask for an opinion.

Table 3.2 Causes of disorders of articulation.

Structural defects	
Tongue	— congenital hypoplasia (small immobile tongue)
	— macroglossia in Hurler's syndrome, Down's syndrome, Beckwith's syndrome
Palate	— cleft palate: often associated with a conductive hearing loss
	— palatal disproportion and submucous cleft
Nasal obstruction	— difficulty with 'n', 'm', 'ng': no air entry when asked to sniff
	— adenoidal enlargement
	— displacement of nasal septum
	— chronic rhinitis
	— partial choanal atresia (rare)
Malocclusion of the jaws	— micrognathia: a small lower jaw with protrusion of the tongue between the teeth in speech. Occurs in association with cleft palate in Pierre-Robin syndrome
	— prognathism: protrusion of the lower jaw
	Malocclusion causes difficulty with the 's' and 's' blend sounds

Muscular defects

Myotonic dystrophy
Facio-scapulo-humeral dystrophy
Myasthenia gravis

Neurological defects

Cerebral palsy	— 50% have defects in articulation
	— spasticity of tongue, lips and palate gives rise to slow laborious speech
	— feeding problems, drooling
	— involuntary movement
	— incoordination of movements
	— associated mental retardation or hearing loss
Nuclear agenesis	— failure of development of the nuclei of the cranial nerves

VISION SCREENING

Early detection of severe visual impairment is important because:
- Some conditions are surgically treatable, e.g. cataract, glaucoma, retinoblastoma
- Many disorders have genetic implications
- Appropriate guidance can be offered to parents, resulting in benefits in terms of development, vision and general health
- Visual failure is occasionally the presenting sign of serious systemic disease

Screening

At birth

By doctor
- Ophthalmoscopic examination for red reflex to exclude cataract, retinoblastoma
- Inspection for congenital abnormalities, e.g. coloboma, microphthalmos

6 weeks

By doctor
- Ask about family history of squint/'lazy eye', visual impairment
- Ask about any parental concerns:
  - Looking at parents
  - Fixating on objects
    Following moving objects
  - Squinting
- Observe visual behaviour:
  - Visual interest in near surroundings?
  - Fixates and follows either side of midline
  - Abnormal eye movements? Squint?
  - Repeat inspection and ophthalmoscopic examination as above

After 6 weeks

All staff
- Take reported squint or abnormal visual behaviour seriously
- Do not use screening procedures to 'reassure' concerned family or staff
- Diagnosis is the job of the ophthalmic department – refer if there are concerns

7–8 months, 18 months

By health visitor
- Ask about family history
- Ask about any parental concerns
- Parents should be given advice on what to look for in normal visual development, and what to do if they are concerned
- Observe for squint or abnormal visual behaviour (during hearing test is a good time)
- Refer to GP or community paediatrician if any concerns

Where parents or health professionals are concerned about possible visual impairment or ophthalmic disease, a referral to an ophthalmologist should be made.

3–4 years
- Value of screening at this age debatable; district policies vary
- Primary orthoptic screening most effective system and should be preferred
- Insufficient evidence to show that treatment of squint and amblyopia is more effective at this age than at school entry

School entry

By school nurse
- Visual acuity, eyes separately and together, using Snellen linear chart at 6 m

- Alternative tests appropriate to developmental age may be used, e.g. Sonksen-Silver Acuity System; matching Snellen letters
- 6/12 or worse in either eye should be referred, preferably to orthoptist if service allows
- 6/9 in either eye merits retesting in 6 months
- Aim is to detect amblyopia or significant refractive errors
- Test should be in quiet well lit room of 7–8 m length. Tests carried out in poor conditions can give false results

8 years

By school nurse
- Visual acuity as above

11 years

By school nurse
- Visual acuity as above, referrals to optometrist
- Colour vision test - e.g. Ishihara plates, with quantitative test for failures such as City University Plates; appropriate career counselling should follow (see below)
- Children and parents should be given written and verbal information on vision, the possible development of myopia, and how to use the services of an optometrist

The value of testing older schoolchildren to detect new cases of myopia is debatable; most can detect deterioration in vision and most attend an optometrist spontaneously.

Assessment of vision in pre-school child
Community paediatricians may be asked to assess children's vision by parents, GPs, health visitors, nursery staff. In all cases:
- Ask about family history of visual impairment, squint
- Ask about any parental concerns
- Observe visual behaviour in relation to developmental level – fixing, following, abnormal eye movements
- Inspect for congenital abnormalities, e.g. coloboma, microphthalmos
- Corneal light reflexes and cover test (see Fig. 3.6) – this is difficult, especially in infants; abnormal test warrants referral, normal test does not exclude a vision problem
- Ophthalmoscopic examination – red reflex, fundoscopy

Vision testing
- Always carry out in the light of developmental level, and taking into consideration any other disability
- Tests of visual behaviour, e.g. following graded objects of different size, hundreds-and-thousands test
  — Can be useful, but need much experience and require careful implementation – there are pitfalls, especially false negative results
- Visual acuity

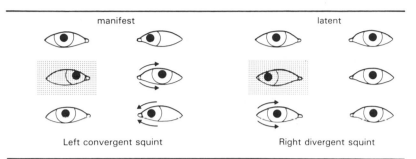

manifest　　　　　　　　　　　　　　　　latent

Left convergent squint　　　　　　　　　　Right divergent squint

Fig. 3.6 Testing for squints. When examining a child for a manifest squint, watch the uncovered eye. When examining for a latent squint watch the covered eye.

- The age of development of normal linear acuity varies – 3/3 vision is achieved by:
    - 20% of 2,5–2,11 year olds
    - 40% of 3,0–4,5 year olds
    - 80% of 4,6–6,0 year olds
- 32% of 5 year olds are unable to name letters
- Linear optotype tests are preferred (e.g. Sonksen-Silver Acuity System [SSAS], or matching letters to Snellen chart) as they are more likely to identify children with significant problems. Children with 6/12 vision on linear optotype tests may achieve 6/9 or 6/6 on single optotype tests
- 90% of 3,0–3,5 year olds and 80% of 2,5–2,11 can match letters on the SSAS
- Eyes should be tested separately where possible
- Tolerance of occlusion increases with age – 90% accept at 4 years
- Standard test distance of 6 m should be used where possible. However, some young children may not be able to comply at this distance, in which case 3 m should be tried

Referrals
- Orthoptist/ophthalmologist
    - Where there are any abnormal findings on examination
    - If there is parental concern about vision
    - Visual acuity 6/12 (or 3/6) or worse in either or both eyes
- A newly recognised paralytic squint at any age merits urgent neurological referral

Colour vision
- 8% of boys and 0.4% of girls have some degree of colour vision defect
- Commonly red–green defects, others extremely rare
- Inherited, but genetics complicated
- Most defects mild but will still fail Ishihara test, which is very sensitive

- Practical problems uncommon – individuals learn to use other clues to compensate, e.g. brightness (saturation); position, as in traffic lights
- No evidence that educational achievement is affected
- There can be problems in school when colour is important, e.g. art, geography, chemistry, electronics – pupils usually sort out these difficulties themselves; exam boards may need to be informed by school
- Only justification for screening is to guide in career choice

Examples of careers where there may be difficulties:
- Quality of product – these careers are likely to be self-selected against
  — Colour matching (e.g. in textiles, printing)
  — Art, design, photography
- Safety reasons, e.g. transport safety lights, colour coding (e.g. electrical components)
  — Armed forces
  — Merchant shipping
  — Railways
  — Civil aviation
  — Police
  — Electrical, electronic, chemical industries
- Usually only certain jobs within a service or industry which may be barred
- Many services and industries make their own assessments, often using trade tests

MANAGEMENT OF THE VISUALLY IMPAIRED CHILD IN THE COMMUNITY

The following areas may need consideration when assessing/reviewing visually impaired children in the community. Clearly not all these can be addressed at once and some themes may be more important than others at different stages. Many of these areas are the professional province of specialist teachers and rehabilitation officers; however, a broader appreciation of the issues involved should help community paediatricians to carry out their own role more effectively.

Medical aspects
- Does the child have ophthalmological review – locally, tertiary centre?
  — Liaison with ophthalmologist regarding diagnosis, treatment, nature of impairment, likelihood and rate of any progression
  — If vision is stable and likely to remain so, the ophthalmologist may feel that follow-up is not justified
  — Is registration blind/partially sighted required?
- Always check hearing – an otherwise mild hearing impairment may constitute a significant disability in a visually impaired child

- Are there any other medical problems/disabling conditions that need to be addressed?
- Has genetic counselling been discussed?
- How good an understanding does the child/family have of the nature and implications of the visual impairment?
- To what extent does the child/family accept the visual impairment and resulting disability? This may be particularly important where progressive conditions are involved. What sources of help are available? e.g.:
  — Counselling services
  — Health professionals
  — Special school staff
  — Voluntary organizations
  — Other families

Development
- Consider whether or not development is appropriate for age, taking into consideration the child's visual impairment
- The visual impairment will make some standard developmental tests unworkable
- Certain areas will normally be delayed in blind children
  — Gross motor skills may be delayed as they tend to be reluctant to explore the environment and they do not have visual positional clues. Sitting and walking may be late
  — Speech may be well developed at the expense of language – phrases are learnt readily but the concepts to which they apply take longer to acquire due to the lack of visual associations; parroting and echolalia may occur
  — The acquisition of social skills, particularly toileting, may be delayed
- The degree of developmental delay depends on the amount of residual vision and on the extent and nature of early developmental and visual stimulation
- If there is concern as to whether or not there is significant developmental delay further specialist assessment should be sought (e.g. using the Reynell–Zinkin scale)

Functional nature of the visual impairment – what can the child see?
An understanding of the child's visual abilities can help in understanding their educational and social functioning.
- What type of things can be seen?
  Size, distance, colour, brightness, background contrast
  — Are lights, windows, the outline of a person or the outline of furniture noticed? (All useful for navigation)
- What are the effects of ambient light conditions, shadows and glare?
- Can facial expressions/body language be seen, and are their social implications understood and used?

- What print features are most useful?
  — Size, colour, contrast, spacing, reading distance
- Other visual features
  — Visual fields
  — Scanning (ability to visually assess the environment)
  — Tracking (ability to follow something visually, e.g. a moving object or a line of print)
  — Photophobia
  — Binocular vision/depth perception
- Variation in visual ability – consider effects of
  — Tiredness, e.g. end of school day
  — General health
  — Progression of condition
  — Appropriate use of aids and glasses
- Interpretation of vision – what meaning is placed on that which is seen? How are visual, auditory and tactile perceptions linked together cognitively? This may be particularly relevant with cortical problems

Mobility
- How does the child manage in:
  — A familiar place?
  — An unfamiliar place?
- Is assistance required, and, if so, to what degree and under what circumstances?
- What dangers need to be guarded against?
- Is a long cane used?
- How much residual vision is there, and is this being used to the full?
- How good is the child's hearing and is this being used to the full?

Educational aspects
- School
  — Mainstream + support
  — Mainstream + vision unit (Individual Needs Centre)
  — Special school
- What is the level of integration?
- Print or Braille user? If a child is likely to change from print to Braille the timing of this needs careful consideration – information on the likely manner and speed of visual deterioration is important here. Tactile and fine motor abilities need to be appreciated
- School environment
  — Classrooms, corridors, steps
  — Lighting
  — Shadows/glare
  — Work surface – angle, distance, colour, contrast
  — Blackboards – clean, colour of chalk, distance and direction
- Aids
  — Glasses – may be tinted

— Magnifiers – lenses, telescopes, closed circuit television (CCTV)
— Brailler – notes may be dictated on tape and Brailled later
— Laptop – voice synthesizer, download to brailler
— Specialist materials – braille translations, enlargements, tactile diagrams
— Talking calculators, clocks etc.
- Medical liaison with school
  — Ophthalmological nature of impairment
  — Discussion of any possible progression
  — Explanation of any other relevant health problems
  — Availability to look into any other concerns staff may have

Blind/partially sighted register
- Registration made on form BD8 by an ophthalmologist
- Register kept by social services team for visual impairment
- Criteria for registration
  — Blind – visual acuity <3/60 in better eye
  — Partially sighted – visual acuity 6/24–4/60 in the better eye
- In practice there may be little benefit to children from registration other than access to certain equipment and resources which some may already be receiving by alternative means

Services review
- The following services may need to be involved if they are not already:
  — Ophthalmologist – local or tertiary centre
  — Orthoptics
  — Low-vision clinic – supplies some visual aids, referral from ophthalmologist
  — Clinical genetics
  — Child development centre
  — Peripatetic teachers for the visually impaired – assess vision; carry out visual stimulation in pre-school children; support children and advise staff in mainstream schools
  — Social services team for the visually impaired – mobility training; maintain register of the blind and partially sighted; access to equipment and resources, e.g. tape libraries; access to other social services resources, e.g. benefits, respite care
  — Voluntary organizations – RNIB; specific societies, e.g. retinitis pigmentosa; local disability groups

Some figures
- The overall incidence of disabling visual impairment in children in the UK is 2–4 per 10 000 births
- 1.6–2.1% of all children are diagnosed as having ocular or vision defect by 2 years
- Mean prevalence of squint is 3.5% for all ages; prevalence much higher in disabled populations

At school entry:
- 96.6% have normal visual acuity
- 2.7% have moderate defects
- 0.6% have severe defects

At age 16 years:
- 8.1% have moderate defects
- 8.0% have severe defects

High-risk groups:
- Low birth weight or infants requiring special neonatal care (increased risk 2.5%, visual impairment more likely to be severe)
- Family history of squint, amblyopia, visual impairment
- Children with other disabilities, e.g. learning difficulties

DISADVANTAGE – CHILDREN IN NEED

- Social factors, such as illegitimacy or low social class, are much more important determinants of educational success than medical factors such as low birth weight
- Definition of disadvantage from National Child Development Study
  Poor housing
  + Low income
  + One-parent or large family

Poverty (EC measure)
- Families whose income is less than half the average for the state
- 4.1 million children in the UK, roughly 1:3, fit this definition

Lone parents
- 1.3 million one-parent families, containing 2.2 million children, roughly 1:5

Poor housing
- 1:12 homes in England are in poor or unfit condition
- In London 1:3 children in local authority or housing association accommodation live in overcrowded conditions
- In 1992, 62 900 households were living in temporary accommodation
- Average figures hide a huge range of variation within a population from 0% in affluent areas to 30% in our poorest neighbourhoods

Other groups to consider include:
- Parents with learning difficulties
- Parents with mental health problems
- Households with a disabled adult or child
- Traveller families
- Those from ethnic minorities
- Unemployment
- Those with overwhelming difficulties
- Children 'looked after' by the local authority and other children living away from their parents

- Young carers:
  - Children and young people who are taking responsibility for the physical care of an adult with a disability; these children often miss school, suffer injuries through lifting, carry out inappropriate personal care tasks, lose sleep, be under emotional stress and lack information or support
- Children not attending school, including those receiving home tuition
- Children excluded from school

Effects (National Child Development Study — NCDS)

Educational
- Three times as likely to display behaviour unacceptable at school
- Five times as likely to be absent from school for 3 months
- Six times as likely to attend a special school for children with moderate learning difficulties
- Seven times as likely to be unable to do basic arithmetical calculation
- Ten times as likely to be unable to read well enough for everyday needs

Medical
- Five times as likely to be incompletely immunized
- More likely to be clinic non-attenders
- Four times as likely to have a hearing loss
- Twice as likely to wet the bed at age 11
- More likely to be admitted to hospital
- More likely to attend an Accident & Emergency department
- More likely to die in childhood

Social
- Twelve times as likely to be in care before the age of 11
- More likely to be on a child-protection register
- More likely to appear before a juvenile court
- Much more likely to be unemployed

Management:

Community level
- Local community profiles should identify disadvantaged areas and lead to positive discrimination in resource allocation
- Within localities, interagency service agreements should ensure that health, education, social services and voluntary groups should provide a service network with local service agreements
- Access to this service should take account of local geography, times of access and language

Early intervention
This consists of:
- Identification as a 'child in need'

- — Health visitor case loads are often divided into low, medium or high intervention, depending upon level of support needed
- Financial help
  - — Advice on budgeting
  - — Advice on benefits – often low uptake of eligible benefits
  - — Provision of help with clothing and other needs
- Advice on
  - — Nutrition (iron deficiency very common pre-school), vitamins
  - — Safety (home, neighbourhood); help with loan, purchase or grant for stair gates, cooker guards, smoke detectors, cycle helmets
  - — Stimulation; play, playgroups, family centres, leisure centres, other community groups and organizations
  - — Health education; smoking, alcohol, mental health
  - — Adult education
  - — Family planning
  - — Family life
  - — Child development and behaviour
  - — This may be achieved by individual or group activities; in clinic or home; through structured programmes such as the Bristol Child Development Programme
- Use of resources
  - — Recreation
    Library
    Toy library
    Leisure centres
    Parks
  - — Child care
    Mother and toddler groups
    Playgroups
    Day nursery
  - — Education
    Nursery school
  - — Local groups
    Cubs or brownies
    Clubs etc.
- Special schemes: family centres
  - — Bristol child care scheme
  - — Use of Open University courses, e.g. 'first years of life'

Keys to management
- Continuity of professional input
- Coordination by 'key worker'
- Recognition that priorities for professionals might not be the same as the family's
- Prevention and education instead of crisis management
- Excellent communication with other workers
- Keeping the service network small

- Partnership with parents
- Regular and planned professional input
- Help rather than criticism

Outcomes
- By early intervention, long-term gains should be expected in:
  — Educational attainment
  — Future employment
  — Health and development

EMOTIONAL AND BEHAVIOURAL PROBLEMS

Emotional and behavioural problems are the commonest cause of disability in childhood. They account for at least 25% of the workload of community paediatrics.

Medical problems that can contribute towards behaviour problems
- Illness in other family members – physical or mental
- Sensory problems, particularly hearing problems
- Clumsy children can have associated behaviour problems
  — May be helped by occupational therapy
- Effects of medication
  — Anticonvulsants, antihistamines
- Temporal lobe epilepsy
- Secondary effects of chronic disease:
  — On the child: sick role; demands and restrictions caused by treatment; unpleasant side effects of treatment; reaction to disability; worry and uncertainty about the future
  — On parents, e.g. on discipline, over-protective
  — On peer group, e.g. teasing, exclusion
  — On teachers, e.g. restrictions, insensitive handling, ignorance, fear
- Unrecognised developmental delay
- Unrecognised general ill health, e.g. chronic infection, anaemia, pain
- Poor control of symptoms
- Language delay:
  — Speech problems leading to communication difficulties are common in the early history of children with behaviour problems
  — This may lead on to learning difficulties and further behaviour problems
- 'Food Allergy':
  — Naturally occurring foods or additives can give rise to hyperactivity which is improved by an exclusion diet
  —Reactions may occur as physiological responses, e.g. to caffeine
- Worry about own health, body image
  — Common in adolescents

Social factors that can contribute towards behavioural problems
- Family discord or breakdown
- Lack of stable relationships
- Frequent moves
- Absence of well defined and consistent rules
- Lack of appropriate model
- Presence and reinforcement of inappropriate models
- 'Parental incompetence'
- Absence of responsible adult supervision
- Physical neglect or abuse
- Sexual abuse
- Solvent and other substance abuse
- Effects of 'video-nasties' and other violent or pornographic materials
- Secondary effect of environmental stress caused by:
  — Poverty
  — Unemployment
  — Poor housing

Educational factors that can contribute towards behavioural problems
- Lack of success, perception of failure
  — May lead to alienation and truancy
- Cultural differences between home and school
- School regime that does not encourage self-discipline, self-esteem, and positive identification of pupils with their school
- Bright but bored

Professional factors that can contribute towards behavioural problems
- Conflicting advice
- Poor communication
- Discontinuity in professional input

Management
First: initial assessment
- Decide whether problem is likely to be self-limiting, e.g. 'normal phase of development', limited in extent, appropriate parental handling
- Decide whether individual intervention by community paediatrician is needed, e.g. rapid deterioration, need for parental support, inappropriate parental response, need to coordinate services, child protection concerns
- Who else needs to be involved and informed? School nurse, health visitor, general practitioner, teacher?
- Decide whether referral to child psychiatric or clinical psychology service is needed, e.g. severe problems, need for behaviour

modification programme, psychotherapy, family therapy, in-patient treatment, deterioration in spite of paediatric intervention

Second: if you decide to take on
- Need a contract of expectations and attendance with family
- Offer to see regularly over a period of time
- Need to ascertain who needs to be seen and in what combination, e.g. parents on own, child on own, parents and child together, grandparents
- Identify and treat any contributing medical factors
- Discuss social and educational factors with appropriate agencies; requires consent; an inter-agency meeting may be invaluable

Thirdly: try behaviour modification approach
- Identify clearly what the unwanted behaviour is
- How often and when does it occur?
- What seems to bring it on?
- What is the parent doing to try to control the behaviour?
  — Diaries kept by parents recording ABC:
      Antecedents
      Behaviour
      Consequences
  — These can help to analyse behaviour
  — Can rules be established for all the family?
- Why is it not working?
  — 'Punishment' is really rewarding the child with attention
  — Inconsistent application
- What are the good things about the child that the parent can praise?
  — Good behaviour can often go unrecognised
- Establish a record of behaviour with rewards, e.g. praise, stars, small sweets for appropriate behaviour, and consistent action, e.g. removal, 'time-out', ignoring unwanted behaviour
- Parents need to know that behaviour initially gets worse before it improves when attempts are made to change it

Fourthly: is the child really the patient?
- Is the child the presenting factor of the parents' emotional problems?
- Are the parents' expectations realistic against the background of normal cognitive and emotional development? For example, accidents are interpreted as naughtiness
- Are the parents over-punitive so that fear of punishment or uncontrolled rage lead the child to go to great lengths to conceal his actions?
- Do the parents have a consistent code of right and wrong, and have they explained it to their children?
- Do parents consistently make threats that they do not mean?
- Do parents encourage self-esteem or self-doubt and humiliation?

Lastly: children need to be forgiven, to have the opportunity to say 'sorry', and to be sure that they are loved
- Established patterns of behaviour may take some time to change
- A sense of humour is often a good substitute for anger

THE DISABLED SCHOOL LEAVER

- The young person leaves the security of school and the paediatric services at much the same time
- Continuity of care can be provided only if the young person and his family are aware of adult services
- Liaison between family and all professionals involved is essential to allow smooth transition
- A medical review well before school leaving may help to bring to light unresolved issues
- Transitional plan review meeting is a good opportunity to discuss future needs with family and relevant professionals

Suggested checklist of issues
- Review young person's understanding of his disability, its cause and implications for the future
- Provision of up-to-date health report for
  — Young person
  — GP
  — Disabled Persons Act officer
  — Specialist careers officer
  — Discuss with young person and parent and give them copies
- Transfer/referral to adult medical services
  — Orthopaedic surgery
  — Neurosurgery
  — Urology
  — Gynaecology
  — Rheumatology
  — Rehabilitation medicine
  — Adult learning difficulties
  — Ophthalmology
  — Hearing services
  — Clinical genetics
- Transfer/referral to adult therapy services
  — Physiotherapy
  — Occupational therapy
  — Speech therapy
- Nursing needs
  — Pressure areas
  — Bowel and bladder care
  — Consider need for community nurse involvement
- Aids

— Artificial limb and appliance centre – chairs, walking aids etc.
— Rehabilitation services
— Low-vision clinic
— Hearing-aid services
- Social services referral
  — Assessment under Disabled Persons Act
  — Adaptations to home
  — Local authority community care arrangements
  — Team for visual impairment
  — Advice regarding local services
- Sexuality
- Review of benefits
- Employment – refer to specialist careers officer; Employment Medical Advisory Service (EMAS) may also be of use
- Review contact with voluntary organizations
- Review leisure activities, holidays and relief care

Disabled Persons (Services, Consultations and Representations) Act 1986 (DPact)

- Sections 5 and 6 require social services departments to assess the needs of disabled school leavers, with a view to providing relevant services
- Social services departments therefore have to decide which school leavers in their area are disabled
- At the first annual review after the 14th birthday of a child with a statement of special educational need the LEA should invite a social services representative with a view to considering whether the child is eligible for assessment under the act. This ought to be done with the knowledge and agreement of the young person and his family
- In DPact, disability is defined in a rather dated manner under the terms of the National Assistance act 1948 'Persons who are blind, deaf or dumb, or who suffer from mental disorder of any description, and other persons who are substantially or permanently handicapped by illness, injury or congenital deformity'. Individual social services departments must interpret this in their own way, and may develop their own more useful criteria for deciding who to assess
- Implementation will vary locally
- Medical reports may be provided, with the young person's consent, to help social services to decide whether or not assessment is appropriate
- The young person does not have to agree to assessment
- Some young people who do not have a statement of special educational need may be eligible for assessment
- It may be relevant to refer young person to the local DPact team before they have a transitional plan
- DPact assessment provides a means of transferring the young person to adult disability services and resources

BENEFITS

This section gives an outline of some of the benefits available to families with children in the UK. The list is not exhaustive and there will be variation with some benefits provided by local authorities. Rates of benefit will change and the structure and regulations are subject to regular review. The information below was compiled in 1995.

Useful sources of information are:

DSS leaflets
- FB2 – *Which Benefit* (in English and Welsh; FB22 in a number of other languages)
- FB8 – *Babies and Benefits*
- HB6 – *Equipment and Services for Disabled People*
- FB31 – *Caring for Someone*
- FB28 – *Sick or Disabled*
- N1 196 – *Benefit Rates*
- Supplies of leaflets available from: HMSO, Oldham Broadway Business Park, Broadgate, Chadderton, Oldham OL9 OJA, and locally at post offices

DSS free telephone advice
- Freeline Social Security – information about social security and national insurance:
  - English   0800 666 555
  - Chinese   0800 25 24 51
  - Punjabi   0800 52 13 60
  - Urdu   0800 28 91 88
  - Welsh   0800 28 90 11
- Benefit enquiry line – confidential service for people with disabilities and their carers:
  - 0800 88 22 00

Help Starts Here – guidance for parents of children with special needs, regularly updated, produced by: Council for Disabled Children, National Children's Bureau, 8 Wakley Street, London EC1V 7QE

Disability Rights Handbook – published annually by: The Disability Alliance, Universal House, 88–94 Wentworth Street, London E1 7SA

After 16 – What Next? – free booklet giving details of services and benefits for young disabled people, available from: Family Fund, Joseph Rowntree Foundation, PO Box 50, York YO1 2ZX

Advice may also be obtained from:
  - Local Social Services
  - Citizens' Advice Bureau
  - Welfare Rights Officers
  - Education Welfare

Some important DSS and NHS benefits

Expectant mothers
- Statutory maternity pay (SMP)
  - Paid by employer
  - There are qualifying criteria
  - Paid for up to 18 weeks
- Maternity allowance
  - For certain people not eligible for SMP (e.g. self-employed)
  - There are qualifying criteria
  - Paid for up to 18 weeks
- Maternity payment
  - Single payment to help buy things for new baby
  - May get it if on income support, family credit or disability working allowance
- Incapacity benefit
  - May be eligible if cannot get SMP or maternity allowance
  - Payable from 6 weeks before to 2 weeks after birth
- Free NHS prescriptions
  - Until baby is 1 year
- Free NHS dental treatment
  - Until baby is 1 year
- Free milk and vitamins
  - Families on income support

Families/children
- Child benefit
  - Non-means-tested weekly payment
  - Children under 16, or under 19 in full-time non-advanced education
- Income support
  - Means-tested benefit for those on low income
  - Personal allowances for each family member, including children
  - Premiums for families with children, people with disabilities, those entitled to ICA, some other groups
  - Help with some housing costs
- Housing benefit
  - Means-tested benefit paid by council to those needing help to pay rent
  - Personal and dependant's allowances
  - Premiums for special needs groups
- Council tax benefit
  - Means-tested benefit to help pay council tax
  - Rules similar to those for housing benefit
- Family credit
  - Means-tested weekly payment for working families on low income

  — Children under 16, or under 19 in full-time non-advanced
    education
- One-parent benefit
  — Non-means-tested weekly payment
  — For anyone bringing up a child alone
  — Paid for eldest child only
- Guardian's allowance
  — Weekly payment
  — May be eligible if bringing up an orphaned child
- Widowed mother's allowance
  — Non-means-tested weekly payment
  — Widows of any age looking after children for whom they get
    child benefit
- Free milk and vitamins
  — Children under 5 in families getting income support
- Reduced-price baby milk
  — Child under 1 not being breast fed in family getting family
    credit
- Free NHS dental treatment
  — Children under 18, or under 19 in full-time non-advanced
    education
- Free NHS prescriptions
  — Children under 16, or under 19 in full-time non-advanced
    education
- Free NHS sight tests and vouchers for glasses
  — Children under 16, or under 19 in full-time non-advanced
    education
- Travel cost to hospital
  — Means-tested benefit
  — If on income support or family credit

Disability
- Disability living allowance (DLA)
  — Non-means-tested regular payment
  — Care component, with three rates of payment, if help
    required with washing, dressing, toileting etc.
  — Mobility component, with two rates of payment, if over 5 and
    have difficulty walking or need supervision/help for safety or
    to find way
- Invalid care allowance (ICA)
  — Weekly benefit for someone caring for disabled person at least
    35 hours a week
  — Disabled person receiving DLA care component at middle or
    highest rate
  — Other qualifying criteria
- Free milk
  — Children aged 5–16 who cannot get to school because of
    disability

- Disability working allowance (DWA)
  — Income-related benefit for those aged 16 or over
  — Have illness or disability that puts you at a disadvantage in getting a job
  — Other qualifying criteria

Some other benefits (local ones may vary)

Local council/social services
- Orange badge scheme (concessionary parking for disabled)
- Concessionary fare schemes
- Day nurseries and playgroups
- Special equipment and home adaptations

Education authority (apply LEA)
- Free school meals – for families on low income
- Free school milk – varies: some to age 7, others to age 11 some only to special schools or on medical recommendation
- Fares to school – varies, usually depending on distance
- Clothing grant – varies, for parents on low income

Disabled person's railcard – British Rail
Family Fund
- Financed by government and run by Joseph Rowntree Memorial Trust
- For families caring for a very severely disabled child living at home and who is under 16, or over 16 in mainstream education and still eligible for child benefit
- A lump sum for specific purposes which arise from care of the child, e.g. laundry equipment, clothing, bedding, recreation equipment, transport; may also help in other ways
- No means test, but socio-economic circumstances are taken into account
- Apply to: Family Fund, PO Box 50, York YO1 2ZX

GENERAL ADVICE TO SCHOOL ON CHILDREN WITH DISABILITIES

- Most teachers in ordinary schools may have little knowledge about childhood illnesses or handicaps
- They may also have much incorrect 'knowledge' or fears about the handicap and be reluctant to take in loco parentis responsibility

The teachers need:
- Careful explanation about the handicap and its effects
- Detailed discussion of the school timetable, highlighting any areas of difficulty
- Practical instruction on any special procedure that the teacher may be required to carry out or supervise, e.g. use of an inhaler

- Recommendation of additional classroom help if the child's needs dictate this
- Offer of on-going support from school doctor and nurse and updating on changes in the child's medical problems
- The child should have a minimum of change to the normal curriculum with emphasis on the needs that are the same as those of the peer group rather than those that are different

4. CLINICAL PROBLEMS IN COMMUNITY PAEDIATRICS

GROWTH

Screening
- The new 9 centile charts should now be used instead of older 7 centile charts
- Measurement of height and weight rightly forms part of most consultations within community paediatrics
- It can, and often does, become a meaningless ritual, performed without precision and for which the original uses have been forgotten
- All children should be screened for growth failure
- In some important causes (e.g. growth hormone deficiency) the child will appear well and in others (e.g. poor growth secondary to social deprivation) the parents are less likely to seek help for themselves
- A suggested framework for screening is:
  — At 18 months
  — Between second and third birthdays
  — At school entry
  — At age 8 if three previous measurements are not available, if there is concern, or if measurement at 5 is below the 2nd centile line
- School nurses or health visitors should refer to the doctor:
  — All children who are below the 2nd centile
  — All children who are crossing centiles
  — Children where there is parental concern
- Height below the 0.4th centile on the new 9 centile charts should always be referred for a specialist opinion

Equipment and technique
General
- Most measurements are made by nurses
- The doctor is responsible with them for ensuring that measurement is accurate, that the results are correctly interpreted and that appropriate actions are taken
- Standardization of equipment using standard weights and a standard rule before any measurements are made, avoids records of apparently shrinking children being recorded
- If measurements are only approximate, where for example, height is

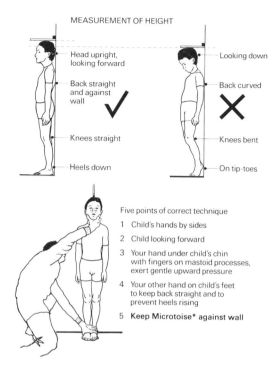

MEASUREMENT OF HEIGHT

Head upright, looking forward

Back straight and against wall

Knees straight

Heels down

Looking down

Back curved

Knees bent

On tip-toes

Five points of correct technique

1 Child's hands by sides

2 Child looking forward

3 Your hand under child's chin with fingers on mastoid processes, exert gentle upward pressure

4 Your other hand on child's feet to keep back straight and to prevent heels rising

5 Keep Microtoise* against wall

Fig. 4.1 Measuring height. Details of the Microtoise portable height measurer are given on page 5

measured by tape measure attached to the wall, then the method must be recorded to avoid errors of interpretation

Length/height
- Children are measured lying down until their second birthday and after that standing up
- All types of equipment consist essentially of a flat surface with a right-angle for recording the position of the head
- Measurements are made without shoes or socks
- Child stands with feet together, flat against the surface, arms by the side and looking directly forwards
- Someone should ensure that the feet remain flat on the ground while gentle pressure is applied upwards from under the mastoid processes (correcting for lumbar lordosis and the slight decrease in height that takes place through the day)

Weight
- Children should be weighed without heavy outer clothing and preferably in vest and pants
- If the child is holding onto a nearby surface, the weight recorded will be too low!

Recording
- As a minimum, the measurement should be recorded both in units and as a centile
- The date is essential as subsequent interpretation will prove impossible if this information is lacking
- Individual charts are desirable for each child's notes
- Growth velocity charts are a useful addition to standard recording:
  — A velocity below the 50th centile means that the child is progressively deviating from normal growth if this pattern is maintained
  — Interpretation can be difficult if measurements are made at intervals of less than a year, as rates can normally vary considerably within this length of time

Interpretation, follow-up and referral
Before this can be done, growth measurements must be supplemented with the following information:

History
- Small for dates?
- Serious events in past medical history?
- Family history of short stature, including parental heights and heights of siblings
- Family history of delayed puberty
- System review with particular reference to:
  — Appetite/dietary problems
  — Chronic respiratory illness
  — Gastrointestinal problems
  — Renal disease
- Adverse social history
- Learning problems and career hopes
- Secondary emotional problems related to stature

Examination
- Lethargy
- Signs of general poor nutrition – e.g. pallor, signs of vitamin D deficiency, wasting
- General physical examination
- Visual acuity (and fields)
- Dysmorphic features
- Disproportion (trunk, limbs)
- Stage of puberty
- Signs of deprivation, e.g. cold hands and feet, passivity or inappropriate affection

Is the child's height compatible with that of his parents?
- The following procedure is adopted:
  — Add heights of mother and father and divide by two
  — For boys, 7 cm is added; for girls, 7 cm is subtracted

- The mean of the adjusted maternal and paternal heights is calculated = mid-parental height
- Mid-parental height is plotted on centile chart at age 19 years
- The child's centile line is followed to age 19 years on the chart
- If the child's centile at 19 years is within 8.5cm for girls and 10 cm for boys of the mid-parental height, then the height is compatible with that of the parents

New charts (Child Growth Foundation)
- These replace the Tanner Whitehouse charts and reflect the changing growth patterns of British children
- Average height has increased over time
- More rapid weight gain in first few months of life then deceleration
- Guidelines and features of the new charts:
  - Have 9 centile lines – each separated by 2/3s of a standard deviation
  - Suggest referral above the 99.6 centile or below 0.4 centile
  - Eliminate the change from lying to standing height measurements at 2 years of age
  - Body mass index charts (weight/height^2) as a reflection of obesity (though increase lean mass, i.e. 'body builders' will also be identified)

Further evaluation
- Most children will not require further investigation and they and their parents can be reassured on the basis of accurate measurements of height and weight, and growth velocity, combined with normal physical examination
- Follow-up is suggested for children whose heights are below the second centile or above the 98th centile and without signs of illness. (This is needed to confirm that the child is growing below and parallel to the second centile)
- Further investigation is needed if:
  - Children are crossing centile lines (it is unusual for children to cross 2 centile lines after the second birthday without good reason)
  - Children are below the second centile and their parents are tall
  - Children have significant findings on history or examination

A suggested scheme is:
- Bone age
- Full blood count
- Calcium, phosphate, alkaline phosphatase
- Urea and electrolytes, creatinine
- Thyroid function tests
- Chromosomes if dysmorphic features present

Causes of growth failure
- The three most common causes of growth failure are:
  - Familial (constitutional), short stature
  - Familial delayed puberty ('short delay')
  - Psycho-social growth failure
- Causes may be conveniently classified by body build:

Short, fat child
- Psycho-social deprivation
- Hypothyroidism
- Panhypopituitarism/isolated growth hormone deficiency (idiopathic, post-cranial irradiation, birth asphyxia, CNS tumour (especially craniopharyngioma), septal optic dysplasia)
- Cushing's syndrome
- Pseudohypoparathyroidism

Short, thin or normal child
- Psycho-social deprivation
- Constitutional/familial short stature
- Familial delayed puberty/maturation delay
- Some low birth-weight infants
- Chronic systemic disease (e.g. cystic fibrosis, chronic renal failure)
- Malabsorption (e.g. coeliac disease, Crohn's)
- Malnutrition from inadequate intake

Short child with disproportion
- Skeletal abnormality, (e.g. achondroplasia)
- Systemic metabolic disorder (e.g. mucopolysaccharidoses)

Short child with dysmorphic features
- Chromosomal abnormalities (e.g. Turners; not all have associated features)
- Other syndromes (e.g. Prader–Willi)

Familial delayed puberty
- More common in boys than in girls
- Family history of late puberty and continuing to grow into the late teens
- Presentation
  - Late in first decade or early teens
  - Not showing adolescent growth spurt
  - No abnormality on examination
  - Delayed puberty
  - Bone age well behind actual age
  - Height plotted for bone age is normal
- Management
  - Counselling and support
  - Follow-up and referral if no sign of puberty or growth spurt by 14 years of age

Psycho-social deprivation
- If records are to be used for medico-legal purposes, measurements should be checked, plotted carefully and signed
- These children show catch-up growth when social circumstances are improved; the converse is also true
- Periods of at least 6 months may be necessary to detect catch-up growth
- Careful examination for the presence of non-accidental injury is necessary

Familial (constitutional), short stature
- Presentation
  - Well child
  - Height centile compatible with parents
  - Not crossing centiles on follow-up
- Caution
  - Some treatable causes of growth failure are inherited, e.g. rare causes of growth hormone deficiency
  - Children in deprived families may have growth compatible with their parents, but be victims of long-term cycles of deprivation

PUBERTY

Stages of puberty
- Puberty is the series of changes that leads to the acquisition of the ability to reproduce
- It is accompanied by endocrine and emotional changes as well as the changes in physical appearance
- Five stages are described
- Stage one is the stage before puberty begins
- There is a wide variation in the age of onset and time needed to pass through all the stages
- Different elements of puberty can develop at different times relative to each other

Boys: genital development
(Ranges quoted are 3rd–97th centile)
- Stage one
  - Testis, penis and scrotum as in early childhood
- Stage two
  - Scrotum and testes grow, skin of scrotum becomes coarser (mean age 12 years: range 10–14)
- Stage three
  - Lengthening of the penis with further growth of the testes and scrotum (mean age 13 years: range 11–15)

- Stage four
  - Penis broadens and glans develops, testes and scrotum are larger and scrotum darkens (mean age 14 years: range 12–16)
- Stage five
  - Adult stage

Pubic hair: both sexes
- Stage one
  - No pubic hair
- Stage two
  - Sparse growth of slightly pigmented downy hair at the base of the penis or along the labia
    (boys: mean 12.5, range 11–15)
    (girls: mean 11.5, range 9–14)
- Stage three
  - Hair darker and coarser, more curled, spreading sparsely
    (boys: mean 13.5, range 12–15)
    (girls: mean 12, range 10–14.5)
- Stage four
  - Hair adult in type but does not include the medial aspect of the thigh
    (boys: mean 14.5, range 12–16)
    (girls: mean 13, range 10.5–15)
- Stage five
  - Adult pattern involving medial aspect of the thighs

Girls: breast development
- Stage one
  - Only nipples are raised
- Stage two
  - Breast bud: breast and nipple raised as a small mound and areola enlarges (mean 11.5, range 9–13.5)
- Stage three
  - Further enlargement of breast and areola but without separation of their contours (mean 12.5, range 10–14.5)
- Stage four
  - Areola and nipple project to form a mound above the level of the breast (mean 13.5, range 11–16)
- Stage five
  - Only the nipple projects

Asymmetrical breast development
- Fairly common during puberty
  - Often a cause of great worry in girls
- Benign and requires reassurance

Gynaecomastia in boys
- Common during puberty
- Causes anxiety, but resolves spontaneously
- Requires reassurance

Menarche
- Mean 13 years, range 11–15. Periods are frequently irregular for the first 2 years

Dysmenorrhoea
- Primary dysmenorrhoea is common and may cause considerable absence from school
- Mefenamic acid 500 mg q.d.s. after food will relieve symptoms and reduce menstrual flow
- Complaints of dysmenorrhoea can represent an oblique way of asking for contraceptive advice

Peak height velocity
- Girls: mean 13, range 11–15
- Boys: mean 14, range 12–16

Delayed puberty
Definition
- A child who has not entered puberty by the age of 14 years in boys and 13.5 years in girls, or a girl of 16.5 years in whom menarche has not occurred

Causes
- Familial delayed puberty
- Debilitating illness
    — e.g. coeliac disease, renal disease
- Syndromes
    — e.g. Turner's, Klinefelter's
- Anorexia nervosa

Effects
- Mainly emotional
    — Feels different from peers
    — Worried that there is something wrong
    — Concern about fertility
    — Usually short and may be treated as if they are younger

Follow-up and referral
- Familial delayed puberty
    — Explanation and reassurance
    — Follow-up to monitor growth and development
    — Refer to section on growth for detailed description
- All others
    — Referral for investigation

Precocious puberty
Definition
- Development of secondary sexual characteristics before the 10th birthday in boys or 8.5 years in girls, or menarche before the age of 10 years

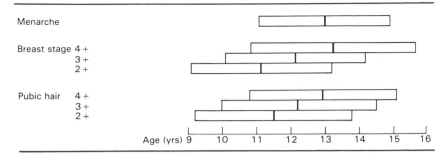

Fig. 4.2 Stages of puberty in girls. The bars show the 3rd, 50th and 97th centiles. thus, 3% of girls have started periods by 11 years, 50% by 13 years, and 97% by 15 years of age (from Tanner & Whitehouse, 1965).

Significance
- Often not due to disease and is more likely to be normal early puberty in girls and where development is just a few months advanced
- Pathology is more likely, e.g. tumour in younger children and in boys

Effects
- Emotional problems due to isolation from peers, and fear of the changes that are taking place
- Development of sexual drive inappropriate to their age
- Clumsiness due to failure to adapt to changes in body build
- Behaviour problems if others have expectations of them beyond their years

Action
- All children require prompt referral for investigation

THE LATE WALKING CHILD

- 97% of children are walking (taking six or more steps unaided) by the age of 18 months
- The remaining 3% can be divided into three groups:
  - 'Idiopathic' late walkers
  - Children with medical problems already identified and which are expected to be associated with delayed gross motor development
  - Children with previously unrecognised problems that come to light because of late walking

'Idiopathic' late walkers
- 93–95% of the late walking children who do not have previously identified disorders fall into this category and can be expected to develop normally

- The following indicators are found commonly:
  - Deviant gross motor development
    Bottom shuffling
    Rolling
    Creeping
  - Other features include
    Hypotonia – especially of the lower limbs
    Late sitting
    Lax joints – back kneeing – poor bulk in legs
    Non-weight-bearing
    Family history of late walking, particularly bottom shuffling
    (said to be more common in Lancashire: hence the name
    Shufflebottom)

Previously diagnosed problems
- The commonest of these will include:
  - Cerebral palsy
  - Other CNS abnormalities
  - Orthopaedic abnormalities
  - Down's and other syndromes
  - Neuromuscular conditions
  - General developmental delay

Newly diagnosed conditions
- Duchenne muscular dystrophy
  - 1 in 3500 male births
  - Diagnosis by serum creatine phosphokinase and muscle
    biopsy
  - Screening all late walking males by CPK would entail testing
    150 boys to find one case
  - There is no treatment, but early diagnosis could prevent
    further cases within the family
- Cerebral palsy
  - Mild or moderate spastic diplegia may present as late
    walking
  - Diagnose by:
    Increased tone (except in bottom shufflers)
    Brisk reflexes
    Difficulty in dorsiflexion of the feet (in contrast to the ease
    of flexion in the 'idiopathic' group)
- Learning difficulty
  - Late walking may be the first indicator of global delay
  - However, gross motor milestones are often reached
    'on time' in children with moderate to severe learning
    difficulty
  - Fine motor and language milestones are far more reliable
    indicators

MOTOR LEARNING DIFFICULTIES – 'CLUMSY CHILDREN'

- Our role
  - Identification of children
  - Then consider referral
  - Or manage with the support of school nurse, occupational therapist, physiotherapist
- Acquisition of motor skills shows a wide variation
- 'Clumsy children' have difficulty learning and performing sequential motor tasks
- Incidence reported to be 5–15% among school children, boys > girls 4:1
- A quarter to a third of these children will have problems in school (1 or 2 children in each primary school class)

Aetiology
- Normal variation
  - Timid temperament
  - Lack opportunity to play and practise
- Isolated delay in motor development
- General developmental delay
- Perinatal asphyxia
  - Insufficient to cause gross neurological impairment
  - Low birth weight
- Hyperactivity
  - Not enough time to perform motor tasks well
- Transient
  - During periods of rapid growth, e.g. adolescence
- Symptomatic (rare)
  - Associated with epilepsy
  - Neuroblastoma
  - Cerebellar tumours
  - Acute cerebellar ataxia
  - Wilson's disease
  - Friedrich's ataxia
  - Hydrocephalus
  - Post chickenpox

Presentation

Gross motor difficulties
- Awkward gait with abnormal foot posture; therefore frequently trips when running
- Poor balance; frequent falls; poor ability hopping or balancing on one leg

Fine motor difficulties
This leads to problems in:
- Self help skills

  — Dressing – buttons, shoes, zips, pullovers
  — Feeding – slow to handle spoon, messy
- Play – jigsaws, bricks, drawing
- School – poor writing

They may also have
- Speech disorder
  — Delayed speech development
  — Developmental articulatory dyspraxia
- Learning difficulties
- Poor visuo-perceptive skills
  — Reading and writing difficulties (letters and numbers reversed and sequences confused)
  — Poor body image
- Behaviour difficulties
  — Particularly the older child, e.g. frustration, social isolation, classroom 'fool', frequent school absence, anxiety, headache, abdominal pain, enuresis
- Laterality may be slow to develop
  — Association with handedness or crossed laterality is not supported

Examination
Note:
- Any hyperactivity
- Emotional immaturity
- Neurological examination to exclude
  — Minimal cerebral palsy
    Hyper-reflexia
    Asymmetry of reflexes
  — Progressive pathology
  — Squint
- Tests of fine motor skills
  — Brick-building
  — Pencil grasp
  — Repetitive fast tapping
  — Finger–thumb opposition fast sequences
  — Pronation–supination
  — Bead threading
- Tests of gross motor skills
  — Standing on one leg
  — Hopping
  — Heel toe walking
  — Skipping
  — Kicking ball
  — Walking on lateral aspects of feet: involuntary mirroring movements of upper limbs (Fog test)
- Movements of muscles involved in speech

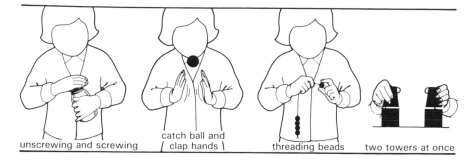

unscrewing and screwing | catch ball and clap hands | threading beads | two towers at once

Fig. 4.3 Example of simple tests for school entrants to identify the clumsy child. Watch for associated movements.

— Blowing
— Whistling
— Tongue protrusion and side-to-side movements

Special tests and equipment

Coffee jar test
- Coffee jar with screw top, five 1-inch wooden cubes with a hole through the centre, a reel, stiff nylon lace
  — Used for screwing, threading, block building, pattern copying

Frostig developmental test of visual perception
- Age range 4–8 years
- Subtests
  — Eye–motor coordination
  — Figure ground
  — Constancy of shape
  — Position in space
  — Spatial relationships
- A remediation programme for individual training is also available

Bender–Gestalt visual motor test
- Copying 10 patterns reveals weaknesses in reproducing spatial relationships

Goodenough draw-a-man test
- Age range 3–15 years
- Score derived from analysis of drawing and can be converted into mental age

Osteretsky test
- Test of postural control and manipulative ability in school-age children
- Child is asked to stand in various positions to test stability and handle objects quickly to test manipulative ability

Weschler pre-school and primary scale of intelligence
- WPSSI: age range 4–15 years

Weschler intelligence scale for children
- Age range 5–15 years
- Separate verbal and performance scales
- Subtests
  - Conceptualization: comprehension; similarities; vocabulary
  - Visuo-motor abilities: picture completion; block design; object assembly
  - Sequencing: repetition of digits; sequencing pictures; coding

Management
- Relieve anxiety and tension for child and family
  - Reassure them that the child is not careless, lazy or dull
  - Usually will improve slowly
- Encourage child in things that he can do well – e.g. swimming, horse riding
- Training can lead to improvement
  - Once a motor skill is learned, it remains
  - A graded series of steps starting with what the child is able to do
  - Aids such as describing the task verbally, as it is performed, may be useful
  - Specialized training – sensorimotor integration
- In planning and carrying out a programme of remediation, the following may be involved:
  - Teacher
  - Occupational therapist
  - Physiotherapist
  - Speech therapist
  - Educational psychologist
  - PE teacher
  - Child psychologist

SPECIFIC LEARNING DIFFICULTY – DYSLEXIA

Definition
- Persistent difficulty in reading, writing, and spelling in comparison with abilities in other spheres, despite conventional education and socio-cultural opportunities
- There is a wide spectrum and degree of difficulty

Incidence
- 2–5% of school children
- Boys > girls; ratio = 3–4:1

Main problems
- Associated with poor visual perception, and poor visuo-sequential memory, and may result in:
  - Reversal and inversion of letters (may also occur as a consequence of immaturity)
  - Mirror writing
  - Difficulty in copying letters
  - Words with letters in wrong order, resulting in bizarre spelling
  - Sequencing difficulties leading to confusion with
    - Days of the week, month order
    - Alphabet
    - Tables
  - Spatial difficulty with poor body image

Associated difficulties
- These may include:
  - Number difficulty (dyscalculia)
  - 'Clumsiness'
  - Left/right confusion
  - Difficulty with time
  - Hyperactivity with poor attention span
  - Emotional problems:
    - May be incorrectly labelled as dull, stupid or lazy
    - Anxious, worried, upset about reading out loud to the class
    - Disruptive
    - Isolated
    - School phobia
    - Abdominal pains
    - Bed wetting
    - Nightmares
    - Tics
    - Secondary to parental anxiety, which will worsen the situation
    - Secondary to the burden of extra work or extra effort
    - But many children, particularly initially, have normal behaviour

Stages at which a child may be seen by a doctor:
Pre-school
- Many children 3–3.5 years of age with specific language delay who speak reasonably well by school entry will subsequently have difficulties learning to read or write
- They are of particular concern if also showing:
  - Delay in perception of shapes
  - Fine motor control difficulties
  - Poor dressing skills
  - Poor drawing skills

Referred from school entrant review
- May obtain history as above
- May present as apparently bright child with intelligent conversation, parents having no worries, but who cannot write name, copy shapes or brick models
- Manifests difficulties with buttons, laces and other fine motor tasks
- Unable to repeat a sequence of digits
- Clumsy in walking and other gross motor skills

Older child failing in school
- Usually seen because of referral for major or associated problems

Scheme for medical evaluation

History
- Family history – frequent family history of reading problems
- Pre-, peri-, post-natal history
    — Placental dysfunction, birth trauma, hypoxia
- Past medical history
    — Epilepsy (possible link between phenytoin use and poor reading ability)
    — Klinefelter's syndrome (delayed speech with later reading and number difficulties)
    — In some sex chromosome abnormalities, e.g. Turner's syndrome, general ability may be within the average range with specific learning difficulties
    — Arrested hydrocephalus
    — Leukaemia with irradiated CNS
    — Severe head injury
- Early developmental history
    — Especially speech and language, gross or fine motor, clumsiness

Physical examination
- This should include:
    — Vision
    — Hearing
    — Neurological examination
        Learning difficulties can predate symptoms by years, e.g. Wilson's disease, Huntingdon's Chorea, some leucodystrophies, slowly growing tumours
        Look for cerebral palsy; motor difficulties may be minor, e.g. abnormal pincer grasp, minor athetoid posturing, tendency to toe walk, brisk or asymmetrical reflexes, limited ankle dorsiflection (41% of children with cerebral palsy showed reading retardation in the Isle of Wight study)

Special diagnostic tests employed by specialist teachers

Aston index
- Test for learning difficulties, particularly with writing, reading and spelling. Designed for children aged 5–14 years. Tests visual, auditory and intellectual function giving an individual profile which can be used to plan a remedial programme

Slingerland screening test
- Gives a profile of perceptual–motor ability which can be used in planning a remedial programme

Boder test of reading and spelling patterns
Dunlop test
- To look for the presence of a fixed reference eye; if not present, occlusion therapy or exercises under the care of an orthoptist may be recommended. However, there is little evidence of benefit

Frostig test of spatial perception

Help available
- Referral to educational psychologist for full assessment of educational needs and provision will usually have been made by the child's school
- Some speech therapists with special interest may be helpful
- Occupational therapist for help with fine motor body image skills
- Physiotherapist for help if clumsy in gross motor movements
- Lap-top computers may be very useful for many children
- Schools can request examination boards to make special allowances in terms of time, spelling concessions, use of word processor. Some will permit pupils to dictate their answers
- British Dyslexia Association
- Parents are often relieved to be told that their child has real difficulties, not just 'overanxious mum' or 'lazy'
- Psychological support, explanations and examples of highly successful individuals who are dyslexic are essential components
- Child's motivation returns with success

ASTHMA

- Asthma is the commonest treatable chronic medical condition of childhood
- Between one in four and one in six children have at least one wheezy attack by the age of four
- Some children with asthma are still diagnosed as having 'bronchitis' or 'chestiness' and receive ineffective treatment with antibiotics
- Most children with asthma improve with age, but they rarely 'grow out of it' by a particular age
- Asthma frequently recurs in later life

Cause
- The underlying abnormality in asthma is an increased bronchial lability
- A large number of triggers can precipitate wheezing and should be identified in individual cases:
  — Allergy to house dust mite
  — Exercise
  — Cold air
  — Pollens
  — Viral infections
  — Emotion
  — Animal fur
  — Atmospheric pollutants, e.g. cigarette smoke
  — Some drugs, e.g. aspirin, ibuprofen
  — Certain food colourings, e.g. tartrazine
  — Some foods/Coca Cola

Risk factors
- Family history of 'bronchitis', asthma or hay fever
- Hay fever or eczema in the child
- Whooping cough or bronchiolitis in early life
- Cystic fibrosis
- Some believe, though objective evidence is lacking, that exclusive breast feeding and exclusion of cows' milk products in early life may prevent asthma. Remember that soya protein can precipitate asthma

Diagnosis and preliminary assessment
History
- Colds going to the chest and persisting for days
- 'Chestiness'
- Night-time cough
- Breathlessness, cough or wheeze on exercise or with excitement

Examination
- Chest shape usually normal:
- Recession of lower ribs or hyperinflation suggests chronic bronchoconstriction
- Auscultation
  — Usually normal between attacks
  — Occasional persistent mild rhonchi or reduced air entry suggests chronic bronchoconstriction

Investigation
- Reduction of peak flow in response to exercise and restoration following administration of a bronchodilator is a useful diagnostic test
- Peak flow measurements are also a good guide to severity
- In younger children in whom peak flow measurements are difficult, a trial of a bronchodilator or regular cromoglycate or inhaled steroid

if there is persistent cough, is often the best way of confirming the diagnosis

Management

Aim
- No restriction on exercise and undisturbed sleep

Precipitants
- It is rarely possible to exclude all precipitants
- Skin testing is often not helpful
- A good history is often invaluable

Exercise
- Should be encouraged and a bronchodilator taken before exercise if necessary

House dust mite
- Trials of meticulous dusting of the child's bedroom are not encouraging, but parents may wish to give it a try
- Intervest covers for mattresses or the cheaper Alputec may reduce dust mite penetration
- Acaricides reduce number of house dust mites but doubtful clinical significance in trials
- Vacuum or clean mattresses/duvets regularly. Wash furry toys

Animal fur
- Discourage acquiring furry pets, but only advise giving away pets if there is a clear association
- Keep pets out of the bedroom

Foods and additives
- It is generally not worth investigating this unless there is very strong suspicion
- Reducing additive intake is harmless
- Any rigorous dietary regimes must be supervised by a dietician

Cigarette smoke
- Strong advice to parents and to the child, when older, must be given

Medication

Bronchodilators (β_2 agonists and theophyllines)
- Can be used for:
  — Acute attacks
  — Prior to exercise
  — Regularly if there is frequent wheeze
- Available as:
  — Syrups for young children who cannot manage an inhaler
  — Tablets, including slow release preparations that are useful at night for prolonged effect
  — Dry powder inhaler from 3–4 years old; it is easy to check whether dose has been taken and is less liable to overuse by older children

— Metered aerosols can be used from adolescence, but can be used by some younger children with help of a 'spacer' device
— Nebulized bronchodilators are used for severe attacks when unable to use inhaler or for very young children

Cromoglycate
- Used for:
  — Prevention of cough and wheeze
  — Exercise-induced asthma
- Must be taken regularly
- Available as:
  — Dry powder inhaler
  — Metered aerosol
  — Nebulizer solution

Steroids
- Used for:
  — Prevention
  — Acute severe attacks
- Must be taken regularly
- Available as:
  — Tablets for acute attacks as a short course; side-effects are not a problem
  — Tablets are only rarely needed for long-term prevention; side-effects can then be a serious problem; management should be supervised
  — Dry powder inhaler ⎫
  — Metered aerosol   ⎬ side-effects are not usually a problem
  — Nebulizer solution ⎭

Management plan (adapted from Thorax 1993:43)
- Start treatment at appropriate step then increase accordingly. Use oral steroids for *acute* exacerbation at *any* step

Step 1
- Occasional use of relief bronchodilators
- Once daily 'as required' β agonist
- Ensure appropriate technique and patient is complying with treatment before going to next step

Step 2
- Regular inhaled anti-inflammatory agent
- Intermittent 'as required' β agonist *and* chromoglycate (20 mg t.d.s. dry powder or metered dose 10 mg t.d.s.)

Step 3
- Inhaled steroids
- Intermittent β agonist and beclomethasone or budesonide (50–200 µg b.d.)
- Consider a 5-day course of oral steroids or double inhaled dose for initial stabilization before starting baseline treatment

Step 4
- High-dose inhaled steroids
- As step 3, but using 400–800 µg daily
- Consider adding twice-daily long-acting β agonist
- Spacers used with metered inhalers improve lung deposition
- Suggest rinsing mouth/brushing teeth after administration to reduce oral absorption
  (N.B. Short-term reduction in tibial growth at above steroid dose. This cannot be extrapolated to the long term)

Step 5
- (a) as Step 4 *and* slow-release xanthines or nebulized β agonists
- (b) addition of regular oral steroids – as step 5(a) with alternate low-dose prednisolone (5–10 mg)
- Consider regular ipratropium or subcutaneous infusion of a β agonist
- May need hospital follow-up

Stepping down
- Regularly review need for treatment
- Stop regular anti-inflammatories after 6–12 months if no/few symptoms
- Use anti-inflammatories for seasonal symptoms only during season

Management in very young children (0–2 years)

Particular problems
- Recurrent wheeze and cough are associated with viral respiratory infections often without a family history of asthma or atopy. Try to reduce passive smoking
- Diagnosis relies on symptoms as opposed to objective lung function tests
- Currently a paucity of suitably designed/tested inhaler devices for this age
- Very few controlled trials of treatment
- Variable response to bronchodilators but they should be tried. Bronchodilator syrups are usually less effective than inhaled treatment and have more systemic side-effects
- Anecdotal evidence suggests ipratropium is more effective than salbutamol under 1 year, but no controlled trial
- The younger the child, the more other disorders may mimic asthma (i.e. gastro-esophageal reflux, cystic fibrosis, inhaled foreign body, congenital abnormalities or chronic lung disease of prematurity
- Nebulized drugs in infancy may paradoxically result in initial bronchoconstriction

General advice
- Normal activities encouraged
- Exercise helpful, especially swimming (prophylactic treatment is needed)

- Patients and parents have relevant understanding of asthma and its management

Follow-up
- Regular follow-up should be undertaken by GP or community paediatrician
- Most children do not require hospital supervision
- Check:
  — Frequency of wheeze (school attendance is a good indicator)
  — Names of medication and when they are taken as well as how often missed; therapeutic intention and reality are often quite different!
  — Diary records of symptoms (day/night); peak flow and medication are invaluable in monitoring treatment
  — Technique, especially with metered aerosols; keep a store of devices and recognise the need to teach and monitor their correct use
  — Chest shape and breath sounds
  — Growth
  — Peak flow

Advice to school
- As asthma is so common, with at least one child in each class, every teacher requires some basic knowledge
- Normal activity should be encouraged and one should stress that with proper treatment, people with asthma can win Olympic gold medals
- Treatment should be available in school, e.g. lunchtime doses, doses before exercise; in most cases, children should carry their own inhalers – this should always be the case in older children
- School doctor should be alerted if attendance is poor or activity restricted
- Parents should be contacted if child becomes severely wheezy
- Teachers need reassurance that children with asthma will not suddenly collapse

Careers advice
- In severe chronic asthma, certain working conditions should be avoided:
  — Polluted or dusty atmosphere
  — Cold and damp conditions
  — Heavy manual work
- In children with few problems, the natural history should be remembered and similar advice given to avoid occupational problems if symptoms return in adult life
- Work with animals should be avoided if this is suspected as a precipitant

ATOPIC ECZEMA

- Affects up to 5% of all children
- In 70% there is a family history of atopy (eczema, asthma, hayfever)
- Resolves by age 5 years in 50% and 10 years in 80%
- Features
  - Itching
  - Weeping vesicular lesions
  - Dry cracked areas
- Distribution
  - Most commonly flexures – wrists, knees, elbows
  - More widespread in severe cases
- Complications
  - Secondary infection (common)
  - Damage from scratching
    Excoriation, bleeding
    Lichenification, pigmentation
  - Emotional problems resulting from:
    Intractable itching, loss of sleep
    Sensitivity to self-image and reactions of others
- Management
  - *Counselling* and information for parents and children, stressing:
    Need for regular therapy
    Use of cotton rather than woollen garments next to the skin
    Use simple soap powders rather than biological ones and fabric conditioners
    Avoid over-clothing and over-heating
  - Recognition and avoidance of aggravating factors, e.g. proven allergies, psychological factors
  - Emulsifying ointment to be used instead of soap
  - *Emollients* added to the bath very helpful with dry lesions
  - Bubble baths forbidden
  - *Topical steroid preparation*:
    Ointment for dry lesions
    Cream for moist lesions
    Weakest effective should be used starting with 1% hydrocortisone
    Fluorinated steroids should not be used long-term and should never be applied to the face. They are particularly useful for acute exacerbations where they can be used intensively (t.d.s) for a limited period, i.e. *one week only*. Follow up these children as some parents may be tempted to continue as they are so effective. *Limit use*
  - Tar-impregnated bandages may be useful to treat and protect chronically scratched lesions
  - Treat itching with an oral antihistamine, particularly at night

- *Antibiotics*
- Topical antibiotics for supradded infection though oral flucloxacillin may be more useful if extensive infection
- *Diet*
- Debatable role. Some are helped by Evening Primrose Oil (oral) or transient exclusion of citrus fruits or dairy products

Advice at school
- Some forms of messy activity, e.g. sand or clay may aggravate eczema
- Swimming is usually not a problem, but children should shower thoroughly afterwards
- Painful flexural lesions can restrict movements in games: perspiration can add greatly to the child's discomfort. Under these circumstances the child should not participate in games lessons until they are healed
- Children are often unhappy to expose their skin to others while changing for games; this problem needs to be handled sensitively

Advice on career
- Occupations in which the hands are kept wet or exposed to irritant substances should be avoided, e.g. hairdressers, motor mechanics

VERRUCAE

- Verrucae and other warts do not need treatment unless they are painful
- Will resolve spontaneously, 65% within 2 years, and will leave an immunity
- Much pupil and nursing time can be lost in unnecessary treatment
- Warts can become painful through over-enthusiastic treatment or secondary bacterial infection
- Exclusion from swimming or covering should not be necessary

Treatment for painful lesions
- Treatment may need to be continued for many weeks
- Peeling and keratolytic agents
  - Contain salicylic acid and lactic acid (e.g. Salactol, Duofilm, Cuplex)
  - Applied at night under a plaster
  - If kept on in the daytime, the skin becomes soggy and painful
  - For keratinous warts, 10% salicylic acid ointment can be used under a plaster and the wart pared down each morning with an emery board
- Formaldehyde and glutaraldehyde solutions
  - For mosaic warts, particularly if associated with hyperhydrotic feet
  - 3% formalin is used as a foot soak for 20 minutes each day (only the sole of the foot)

- Proprietary glutaraldehyde preparations can be painted on warts if they are few in number (e.g. Glutarol, Verucasep)
  - Less effective on keratotic warts
- Silver nitrate
  - For solitary warts on non-weight-bearing surfaces
  - Do not use more than twice a week
- Liquid nitrogen
  - Rapidly effective
  - Painful
- Secondary infection
  - Daily potassium permanganate soaks
  - Topical chlortetracycline

RASHES ON BABIES

Spots that will disappear
Parents can be reassured on all of the following:

Capillary naevi or stork marks
- Small dilated capillaries usually on eyelids, forehead, or nape of the neck

Strawberry naevi
- Raised, bright red lesions
- Usually appear shortly after birth and grow over the first few months of life
- Go pale in the centre and gradually resolve
- Rarely, very large naevi can cause problems by bleeding, or pressure effects giving rise to distorted growth or amblyopia by preventing eye opening

Mongolian blue spots
- Confluent flat bluish pigmentation, usually found in the sacral area
- Commonly seen in babies of African or Asian origin, but can be found in others
- Usually disappear by the end of the first decade
- Must not be confused with bruises

Milia
- Tiny yellow-white spots seen on the face of the newborn

Erythema neonatorum
- Widespread erythema, sometimes papules and pustules
- Must be distinguished from staphylococcal infection, which is more likely if skin creases are involved

Areas of depigmentation at sites of previous trauma, infection or inflammation
- Occur on pigmented skins and will resolve, but slowly

'Non-specific' rashes
- Many babies in the first year of life have rashes which, at least to the non-dermatologists, are non-specific

- They are often seen on the face and loosely described as heat rashes

Spots that will not disappear and which may require treatment

Ammoniacal dermatitis
- Widespread erythema in the napkin area with ulcerated lesions
- Does not involve the flexures
- Treatment:
  - For mild cases:
    Frequent nappy changes to prevent urine being left in contact with the skin
    Careful washing of the bottom at each nappy change
    Terry Nappies
    Use of a nappy liner
    Use of a proprietary cream (often barrier creams or weak acids to neutralize ammonia released by bacterial breakdown of urea.) Rinsing nappies in a solution of one tablespoon white vinegar to a gallon of water has the same effect
  - For more severe cases
    Leave exposed
    1% hydrocortisone topically
    Look for and treat secondary infection (fungal or bacterial). Maybe fungal, so look for oral thrush

Monilia
- Bright red erythema in the napkin area, spreading from the anus and involving the flexures
- Look for and treat oral lesions with nystatin suspension and skin lesions with nystatin ointment
- If co-existent ammoniacal dermatitis, combination of nystatin and hydrocortisone is useful
- If recurs following treatment, suspect monilia in mother and treat if found

Seborrhoeic dermatitis
- Erythematous greasy yellow lesions found in the napkin area, behind the ears, on the scalp (cradle cap), forehead and eyelids
- Treatment unnecessary in mild cases
- Topical hydrocortisone is effective, but may be needed in combination with nystatin or an antibiotic as secondary infection is common
- For cradle cap 'traditional' remedies such as washing the hair in a solution of one teaspoon of sodium bicarbonate in a pint of water, followed by olive oil, and gently rubbing off the scale the following morning, are usually effective, as are 'over-the-counter' cradle cap shampoos

Ichthyosis
- Autosomal dominant condition often associated with eczema
- Dry skin resembling fish scales
- Treat with generous applications of emulsifying ointment

Staphylococcal skin infections
- Pustules
- Should be treated with systemic flucloxacillin in young babies

Eczema
- See separate section in text

ACNE

Should always be treated sympathetically as even the mildest cases can cause great anguish to the adolescent.

Cause
- Increased sebum production
- Colonization of sebaceous glands by bacteria
- Infants: if severe, consider androgen secreting lesion
    - Causes
        Increased sebum
        Colonization
        Drug therapy with systemic steroids and some anticonvulsants
        Occasionally by occlusion (i.e. laceration and friction by head bands, collars)

Lesions
- Blackheads
- Comedones
- Spots
- Nodules
- Cysts
- Scarring

Mild cases (blackheads and spots on face)

Management
- Do not squeeze
- Topical therapy
    - Exfoliants, e.g. benzyl peroxide
    - Cause redness and peeling, which removes lesions
    - Start with 2.5% jelly, increasing to 5 or 10% as tolerance increases
    - Fair-haired individuals are less tolerant
    - Apply at night and wash off in the morning
    - Soaps
        Useful degreasants
        e.g. Nutrogena acne soap

Moderate cases (cysts on face, back and chest) and mild cases in which treatment has failed

Management
- Topical therapy (if accepted)

- Tetracycline (is preferentially concentrated in pilosebaceous units and absorption is impaired by coexistent iron therapy or milk) or erythromycin
- 1 g/day before breakfast for 3 months
- Improvement after 6 weeks
- No place for half-hearted treatment
- May relapse later and need further 3 months' treatment
- May improve in natural sunlight
- Dietary manipulation not medically proven, but alternative medicine suggests specific diets low in fats/additives with higher fibre and fluid

Severe cases (multiple cysts, pits, scars and keloids) and moderate cases in which treatment has failed

Management
- Refer to dermatologist
- Treatments available:
  - High-dose clindamycin
  - Isotretinoin – vitamin A analogue
  - Hormone treatment
    These treatments have a high incidence of unpleasant side-effects, but complete cure is possible in 4–6 months

FITS

Classification
- Partial
  - Generally without loss of consciousness
    (a) sensory (i.e. abdominal pain)
    (b) motor (i.e. focal myoclonic jerks)
    (c) complex (i.e. repetitive, uncharacteristic behaviour)
  - Previously temporal lobe epilepsy
- Generalized
  - Impaired consciousness and often symmetrical bilaterally without local onset
    (a) tonic clonic (previously grand mal)
    (b) absence (previously petit mal)
    (c) infantile spasms, atonic, tonic or clonic
- Unilateral
- Unclassifiable

Neonatal
- Occur in 0.5% of neonates
- Often minimal signs, e.g. flickering eyes, head turning, colour change, twitching limbs
- Associated with:
  - Birth trauma/asphyxia

— Meningitis
— Intracranial bleed
— Metabolic abnormalities, e.g. hypoglycaemia, hypocalcaemia
- All suspicious cases must be referred to hospital
- Prognosis is often, though not invariably poor
- Hypocalcaemic fits and benign familial neonatal fits have a very good prognosis

Infancy

Tonic clonic
- May not be associated with loss of consciousness and diagnosis may be difficult as in neonatal fits

Infantile spasms
- Sudden flexion or sometimes extension of the body singly or up to several times a minute
- Associated with characteristic EEG findings (hypsarrhythmia)
- High risk of underlying problem, e.g. meningitis, metabolic abnormality, cerebral structure abnormality
- Generally very poor prognosis (but better for idiopathic cases)
- Must all be referred urgently for hospital investigation

Older children

Febrile convulsions
- Common, affecting one in thirty children and often familial
- Occur between 6 months and 5 years of age
- About one in three have a recurrence of fits
- Long-term sequelae are rare, though a few go on to have temporal lobe epilepsy if convulsions are prolonged
- Admission to hospital is necessary if serious infection, e.g. meningitis, cannot be excluded or parents are very anxious and for the first febrile convulsion
- Follow-up involves reassurance of parents (many believed their child would die), antipyretic advice (Paracetamol or Ibuprofen), appropriate clothing and not overcooling the skin by tepid sponging as this caused peripheral vasoconstriction, and advice on handling future febrile episodes
- When to call ambulance (usually after 10 minutes of continuous tonic/clonic movement)
- Advice on using home rectal diazepam if recurrent febrile convulsions

Generalized tonic clonic
- Sudden loss of consciousness and motor control, with or without aura
- Child falls, limbs jerk, breathing irregular and may turn blue
- Prognosis depends upon presence of associated problems, e.g. cerebral palsy

- Long-term outlook is often good, particularly for isolated or infrequent fits and for those that only occur at night

Generalized absence
- Easy to miss
- Child momentarily stops what he is doing, eyelids may flutter, looks blank; after a few seconds he may carry on where he has left off
- Can occur many times an hour and be very disruptive
- Long-term outlook is very good as there are generally no associated problems

Complex partial
- Wide variety of fit, e.g. head turning, lip smacking, limb movements or a variety of body sensations such as smell, taste and abdominal pain
- Generally no loss of consciousness or falling
- Specific learning difficulties, mental handicap and behaviour problems occur more commonly than in other types of epilepsy
- Many continue to have fits in adult life
- Social adjustment in adult life may be poor
- Generally no loss of consciousness (i.e. falling) though may have impaired consciousness (not with it)
- Ask about associated autonomic phenomena (pallor/flushing) or facial asymmetry during attacks

Focal epilepsy
- Rare in childhood and suggests focal lesion
- Outlook is that of the underlying problem

Partial motor
- Very brief loss of motor control
- Child may appear to stumble or fall forwards
- Can occur many times in an hour
- Often associated with other neurological problems and outlook is often poor

All children with fits require referral for assessment with the exception of an isolated grand mal fit or febrile convulsion.

Prescription for immunizations will need to be reviewed; this is classified as a *special consideration* not a *contraindication*.

Is it a fit?

At the initial assessment the following need to be differentiated:

Normal baby movements
- Watch baby with mother present

Jitteriness
- May be associated with hypoglycaemia or hypocalcaemia but can be a normal finding. Not associated with abnormalities of gaze/eye movement and is very stimulus sensitive unlike seizures

Breath holding
- Precipitated by frustration or fright
- Quick recovery

Faint
- Situation conducive to faint, e.g. prolonged standing in a warm room
- Light headedness and pallor prior to collapse
- Quick recovery
- Incontinence and twitching can occur during a faint, especially if not lain down

Nightmares and night terrors

Colic in infants

Less common differential diagnoses include:
- Reflex anoxic seizures (vagal attacks)
  — Generally under 2 years
  — Often a precipitating factor, e.g. minor trauma or a fright
  — Child falls suddenly, looks pale and floppy for 1–2 minutes
- Cardiac arrhythmias
  — Rare
  Often occurs during exercise
- Migraine
  — Neurological deficits may occur during initial vasoconstrictive phase
  — Headache is occasionally not present
- Hysterical attacks
  — Can be very difficult to differentiate
  — Hyperventilation may produce symptoms
- Behaviour disorder
  — Episodic aggressive and destructive behaviour may be confused with epilepsy (fits of temper)
- Benign paroxysmal vertigo
  — Generally between 3 and 5 years
  — Child is unable to stand and appears frightened
  — May have pallor, nystagmus, sweating and vomiting
- Metabolic problems
  — Recurrent hypoglycaemia
  — Chronic hypocalcaemia

Investigation
- Diagnosis of epilepsy is mainly on clinical grounds. *Imperative to get clear history*
- The following investigations may be useful in confirmation of the clinical diagnosis or in determining aetiology:
  — EEG

Diagnostic in many types, e.g. generalized absence, infantile spasms
— Fasting blood sugar and calcium
— Metabolic screen, particularly where epilepsy occurs in early life
— CAT scan where a focal lesion is suspected

Advice to schools

- Single fit or night-time-only fits
  — No restrictions necessary
- Recurrent fits
  — In schools the headteacher takes the final decision on any restrictions, but will need professional advice
  — Parents as well as teachers need to be involved in the decision
  — Restrictions will depend on the frequency and severity of the fits and the likelihood of an injury if a fit occurs
  — Swimming should be encouraged, but individual supervision may be recommended
  — Woodwork and laboratory work would usually not present a risk if normal safety precautions are used
  — Climbing heights may need to be restricted, but each case should be considered independently
  — It is vital to emphasise that the child should be treated as normally as possible
  — Teachers may have many fears and misconceptions about the condition and need advice on issues such as:
    Management of a fit
    Effects, if any, on learning
    Maintenance of normal expectations with regard to progress and discipline
- Medication
  — Only rarely causes drowsiness more than temporarily
  — If fits or medication are thought to be affecting the child's progress at school, this should be reported and a review arranged

School leavers

- If reasonable, a trial of stopping treatment should be attempted well before school leaving so that a recurrence of fits does not affect the chance of getting a job or a driving licence
- Regulations will preclude some occupations, e.g. driving some types of vehicle even where there is only a past history of a fit
  — It can be an offence for a job applicant not to disclose this information
- Advice will depend upon the type and severity of the fits
- Driving, working at heights and with machinery are the most common areas of difficulty

- Expert advice should be obtained from the specialist careers officer, unless fits only occur at night. Parental consent is necessary for the referral to be made. The young person whose future it is, is central to any discussion

JUVENILE ARTHRITIS

Onset types (within 3 months of disease onset)
- Pauci-articular – four or fewer joints
- Polyarticular – over four joints
- Systemic – those with fever, rash and arthritis

Associated features

Pauci-articular onset
- Most common type
- Predominantly young girls
- Associated with positive ANA (antinuclear antibody)
- Risk of chronic iridocyclitis, especially if ANA+ve. This is asymptomatic and is detected by slit-lamp examination. Complications leading to blindness include glaucoma and cataracts
- Generally good outcome
- Knees, ankles, wrists and neck most commonly involved

HLA B27-related arthritis
- Often starts with a few joints involved
- Commonly knee involvement with the development of hip, sacro-iliac, back and small joint involvement
- Occurs in older boys
- Family history of ankylosing spondylitis, psoriasis, ulcerative colitis, Crohn's disease, Reiter's disease
- Risk of acute iritis (symptomatic red eye)
- Often persists in adult life

Polyarticular
- Seronegative
  — Rheumatoid factor-negative
  — Occurs in girls and boys
  — Symmetrical arthritis
  — Generally good prognosis
- Seropositive
  — Juvenile rheumatoid arthritis
  — Rheumatoid factor-positive
  — Rare disease occurring in adolescent girls
  — Aggressive erosive disease
  — Systemic disturbance: anaemia and weight loss
  — Joint replacement may be needed in adolescence

Systemic disease
- Girls and boys all ages

- Fever, weight loss, rash, anaemia, arthritis
- Differential diagnosis infection and malignancy
- Systemic features usually settle
- Arthritis can appear late (1 year from onset)
- Can have progressive destructive arthritis
- Variable outcome

Management
- Aim to maintain function, posture and growth
- Daily home exercise programme
- Formal physiotherapy and hydrotherapy
- Splints for work and resting, night hip traction
- Maintenance of mobility
  — Bicycles, swimming
- Drugs
  — Anti-inflammatory: naproxen, ibuprofen
  — Antipyretic: ibuprofen, paracetamol
  — Disease-modifying: methotrexate, sulphasalazine, chloroquine, gold, penicillamine, corticosteroids (oral or pulse intravenous)
  — Eye drops: corticosteroids, beta-blockers
- Diet
  — Drugs and illness may cause anorexia
  — Avoid obesity
- Clothing should be designed to allow independence

Advice to school
- Almost all children can be placed in mainstream education with appropriate support
- Physical and emotional independence must be encouraged
- Disease activity may fluctuate
  — Do not label a child lazy on bad days
  — A child on alternate-day steroids may always alternate a good with a bad day
- Behaviour changes or poor concentration may be a drug problem – especially indomethacin or salicylate toxicity
- Allow children to wear footwear or clothing that maintains their independence (e.g. trainers with velcro fasteners)
- Allow to bicycle to and around school if walking is restricted
- Check that seating and table are appropriate for the child – a tilted table may be necessary if there is neck involvement
- Handwriting may be slow and untidy
  — Consider an electric typewriter or word processor
  — Write to the examination boards to allow dispensation for the degree of handicap
- Involve child in games lessons, e.g. as umpire if unable to participate. Encourage swimming, bicycling, static exercises. Contact and competitive sports may be discouraged

- With motivation, the majority of children with arthritis can lead an independent adult life

MONARTICULAR ARTHRITIS – SWOLLEN JOINT

Presentation
- In older child: swelling, difficulty using joint, discomfort
- In young child: parents notice swelling, tendency to prevent weight bearing, disinclination to use limb

Investigation
- Early diagnosis and treatment may prevent serious, persistent sequelae

History
- Trauma
- Infection
- Recent immunization (rubella)
- Systemic illness
- Travel
- Family history (arthritis, psoriasis, colitis, iritis)

Causes
- Trauma
- Mechanical problems
- Infections
  — Septic arthritis or osteomyelitis, reactive arthritis (e.g. *Yersinia* colitis), as part of a systemic illness such as rubella
- Juvenile chronic arthritis
- Juvenile arthritis (HLA B27-related)
- Blood dyscrasias
- Neoplasms
- Synovial abnormalities

Urgent management
- If the joint is hot and tense with guarded movement, and the child is febrile, then a diagnosis of septic arthritis should be assumed with immediate investigation and intravenous antibiotics
- If pauci-articular juvenile arthritis is suspected, slit-lamp examination is needed to detect iridocyclitis which is asymptomatic until complications ensue

HYPERMOBILITY SYNDROME

- Generalized joint laxity is not uncommon
- It is only rarely associated with generalized disorders such as Ehlers–Danlos syndrome, Marfan's syndrome and disorders of amino-acid metabolism

Symptoms
- Occur in young girls and boys, but predominantly in the pubertal girl
- Frequently occur in athletic children, especially those good at gymnastics
- Often occur during a rapid growth spurt
- Joint pain occurs after exercise and at night
- Knee pain is the most common, but can occur in ankles and upper limbs
- Joint swelling can occur especially in the knees and ankles

Examination
- Both of patient, siblings and parents
- Usually more than one family member is hypermobile
- Ability to extend knees and elbows more than 10 degrees
- Excessive passive dorsiflexion of the ankle
- Passive hyperextension of the fingers, especially the fifth

Management
- Reassure that symptoms improve post-puberty
- Reassure that it is not a deforming arthritis
- Encourage maintenance of muscle strength
- Do not ban sports – let the child restrict himself
- Analgesia can be given – ibuprofen
- Knee pains can be helped by wearing a small wedged heel rather than a flat shoe, to prevent hyperextension
- Sorbothane insoles and supportive shoes

BIZARRE GAITS

- This may be a true conversion hysteria or an exaggeration of a previous organic problem
- These children do not usually have a background of psychological abnormality

Diagnosis
- Bizarre gait that does not fit into any organic pattern
- Disability out of proportion to objective findings
- Evidence of disturbed family psychodynamics (these are not always apparent)
- History of significant life event

Management
- Make the diagnosis and discontinue investigations
- Team work with psychological support and help from the rehabilitation department
- Tackle precipitating or aggravating psychological stresses at school or home

- Give the child and family reassurance on the good prognosis; complete recovery can be achieved
- Give the child an excuse for getting better, e.g. an intense physiotherapy regime
- If symptoms have persisted for weeks, then instant recovery is unlikely; plan a programme with an appropriate period of recovery

BACK PAIN

- An uncommon symptom in children
- Inferred in infants who are unwilling to stand, walk or be carried
- More common in teenagers

Causes over the age of 10 (more common)
- Sports injury
- Postural – examine seating especially in the tall child
- Osteochondritis
- Infection – vertebral or disc space
- Spondylolisthesis
- Disc prolapse
- Osteoporosis – idiopathic, iatrogenic, Cushing's syndrome
- Bone tumours – benign or malignant (primary or secondary)
- Juvenile ankylosing spondylitis
- Spinal cord tumour
- Psychological – physical disease must be excluded

Causes under the age of 10
- Persistent back pain must be investigated urgently to exclude serious underlying pathology

Malignant tumours
- Primary: Ewings, osteogenic sarcoma
- Secondary: neuroblastoma, leukaemia, lymphoma

Benign tumours
- Eosinophilic granuloma, osteoid sarcoma, aneurysmal bone cyst, osteogenic fibroma

Examination
- Assess posture, mobility and gait
- Examine back, legs and abdomen (when undressed)
- Include a full neurological examination

ORTHOPAEDIC PROBLEMS

Intoeing: causes

Metatarsus varus
- Adduction of forefoot in relation to hindfoot
- Most correct spontaneously by eighth birthday

- Refer if adduction is rigid and cannot be passively corrected or if there are neurological signs

Medial tibial torsion
- Outward bowing of the tibia associated with medial tibial torsion, i.e. patella points outwards if the feet are placed in the neutral position
- Most resolve by the fifth birthday

Anteversion of the femoral neck
- Internal rotation of the hip is increased from about 50 to over 90 degrees
- External rotation is reduced
- Patellae point inwards
- Most resolve by eighth birthday
- Those that persist usually have minimal functional disability (osteotomy can be performed if necessary)

Out toeing: causes

Retroversion of the femoral neck
- External rotation increased to over 90 degrees
- Internal rotation minimal
- Most resolve by the age of 2

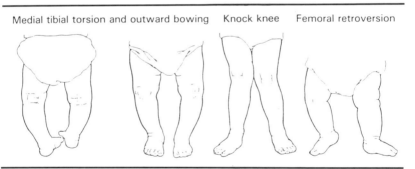

Medial tibial torsion and outward bowing   Knock knee   Femoral retroversion

Fig. 4.4 Orthopaedic problems.

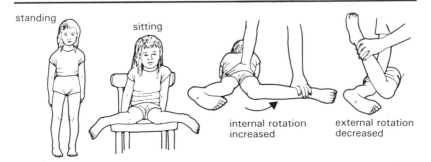

standing   sitting   internal rotation increased   external rotation decreased

Fig. 4.5 Anteversion of the femoral neck, standing, sitting and clinical demonstration.

- Refer if there is associated neurological abnormality

Knock knees (genu valgum)
- Usually resolve spontaneously
- Intermalleolar distances of up to 10 cm can resolve
- Differentiate from rickets
- Persistent cases can be corrected by osteotomy in later childhood

Flat feet (pes planus)
- The medial arch of the foot rests on the ground in the weight-bearing position
- Valgus soles and exercises are unnecessary
- Suitable supportive footwear can reduce excessive shoe repairs
- Flat feet are pathological if the foot is rigid or painful and if the medial arch is not restored by standing on tip toe
- Consider neurological causes such as cerebral palsy or Marfan's syndrome, or congenital vertical talus

COMMON SURGICAL PROBLEMS

Hernia

Umbilical hernia

Problem
- A skin covered spherical protrusion from the umbilicus
- It reduces readily on pressure and the neck is a thick-edged circular ring

Management
- Common in the newborn, with most resolving spontaneously during the first year of life
- Discourage strapping of the hernia
- Refer if not resolved by 4 years of age

Para-umbilical hernia

Problem
- A skin-covered conical protrusion usually just above the umbilicus but occasionally below
- Occurs through a split in the linea alba immediately adjacent to the umbilicus
- The neck is a transverse, elliptical, thin-edged slit

Management
- Occasionally resolves spontaneously if small
- Otherwise refer for repair at age 4 years

Inguinal hernia

Problem
- A lump that comes and goes in the groin
- It is due to persistent patency of the processus vaginalis and may contain bowel or omentum

Examination
- It is impossible to get above the swelling
- If the hernia is not present when the child is examined, a thick cord may be felt on the side that the lump appears

Management
- Refer immediately for elective herniotomy in view of the high incidence of strangulation, especially in younger children

Complications
- The swelling may appear suddenly and be irreducible, or a previously reducible swelling may become irreducible
- Emergency admission for surgery is required

Umbilical granuloma

Problem
- A small ball of granulation tissue at the umbilical cord stump, producing a slight but persistent discharge

Management
- Application of silver nitrate stick, repeated if necessary; warn parents that granuloma will turn black, and protect surrounding skin e.g. with vaseline

Problems of the testes and prepuce

Torsion of the testis

Problem
- A volvulus of the testis on the spermatic cord with interference to the blood supply to the testis

Presentation
- Presents with pain, and on examination, there is swelling, redness and acute tenderness around the testis

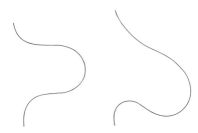

Fig. 4.6 Different contours of umbilical (L) and para-umbilical (R) hernia.

Management
- Refer immediately for surgery
- The opposite testis should be fixated at a second operation to prevent torsion on the opposite side

Disorders of the prepuce
- At birth the prepuce is firmly adherent to the glans
- By the third birthday the prepuce can usually be retracted (90%)
- If it is not, then this can usually be accomplished by gentle manipulation in the bath (if the meatus is visible, then this is all that is needed and circumcision is not necessary)
- Circumcision is needed for phimosis and paraphimosis, a scarred prepuce following balanitis or forcible retraction, or a non-retractile prepuce in which the meatus cannot be seen

Ammoniacal dermatitis of the prepuce
Problem
- An oedematous, red, scaly, and sometimes ulcerated prepuce due to ammoniacal dermatitis

Management
- As for ammoniacal dermatitis of the perineum
- Circumcision is contraindicated

Phimosis
Problem
- Stenosis of preputial orifice, usually acquired secondary to balanitis, ammoniacal dermatitis or forcible retraction, which leads to scarring, but can be congenital

Presentation
- May be asymptomatic or present as slow, dribbling or spraying micturition with ballooning of the prepuce, urinary retention, recurrent balanitis or paraphimosis
- The meatus cannot be seen and, on protraction (attempting to open the orifice by lateral stretching), the preputial orifice does not open up

Management
- Refer for circumcision as all cases will eventually become symptomatic

Paraphimosis
Problem
- Forcible retraction of a moderate phimosis causes the prepuce to be trapped in a retracted position

Management
- Needs referral to hospital
- Might be reduced with pressure from an adrenalin soaked gauze; otherwise dorsal slit

- Circumcision should follow

Balanitis

Problem
- Inflammation arising in the coronal sulcus of the preputial sac

Presentation
- Discharge of pus from preputial meatus without dysuria
- Or may progress so that oedema blocks the preputial orifice with resulting urinary retention

Management
- Warm baths 4–5 times daily may relieve symptoms
- Local or systemic antibiotics may be needed depending upon severity
- If recurrent, refer for circumcision – a limited dorsal slit may occasionally be needed in the acute phase

Hydrocele

Problem
- A scrotal swelling due to a very narrow persistent processus vaginalis

Examination
- Communicating hydrocele will change in size – non-communicating hydrocele will not alter in size with change in posture overnight

Management
- Non-communicating hydroceles will resolve spontaneously
- Communicating hydroceles require surgery
- Sudden appearance of a hydrocele in an older child, in the absence of a good history of trauma, requires urgent referral to exclude a testicular tumour

Undescended testes

Problem
- One or both testes not palpable in the scrotal sac
- The testis is not fully descended unless it can be palpated at the base of the scrotum 4 cm below the pubic tubercle

Assessment
Can be divided into four groups:

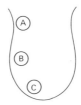

Fig. 4.7 The value of simple drawings to illustrate testicular descent.

- High, but within the scrotum
  — Felt within the scrotum but cannot be brought right down by any manoeuvre
- Retractile
  — Can be brought down to the bottom of the scrotum by gentle massage downwards along the line of the inguinal canal
  — Beyond infancy, examination in the squatting position often allows a retractile testis to descend into the base of the scrotum
- Arrested along normal path of descent
  — 20% of truly undescended testes
- Ectopic
  — Testis has passed normally through the superficial inguinal ring, but then does not follow the normal line of descent
  — 80% of truly undescended testes
  — Sites of ectopic testis in order of occurrence: superficial inguinal pouch, femoral triangle, perineum, pubic area

Management
- Both testes felt in the scrotum 4 cm below the pubic tubercle:
  — No need to re-examine as testes will stay there
- Both testes in the scrotum, but less than 4 cm below the pubic tubercle:
  — Record position of each testis on a simple diagram and follow up
  — These incompletely descended testes may subsequently be absent from the scrotum, or remain high and require referral for orchidopexy or fixation
- One or other testis absent from the scrotum:
  — Refer for orchidopexy from the age of 3 months and certainly no later than 1 year of age, after which spontaneous descent will not occur
  — Orchidopexy is then performed around the age of 2 years
- Late diagnosis and treatment impairs spermatogenesis; testicular tumours are not likely to be diagnosed early if the testis is not in the scrotum

Lumps in the neck

Lateral lumps
Lymph node
- Usually palpable along anterior border of sternomastoid as smooth, firm, rounded swelling in subcutaneous tissue
- If non-mobile or atypical in other ways, refer

Branchial cyst
- Smooth, unilocular, fluctuant, transilluminable swelling beneath anterior border of sternomastoid

- Refer for excision

Lymphangioma
- Soft, multicystic, brilliantly transilluminable, ill-defined swelling
- Refer for excision

Haemangioma
- Ill-defined mass with overlying patch of blue or red skin, emptying partially on pressure
- Refer for assessment

Sternomastoid 'tumour'
- Firm, smooth, ovoid mass, 2–3 cm in diameter, attached to sternomastoid and due to a localized fibrotic nodule
- Role of physiotherapy is controversial
- Rarely surgery is required

Mid-line lumps

Lymph node
- Less common than laterally

Dermoid cyst
- Smooth, firm, unilocular, rounded swelling, subcutaneous or subfascial and usually immediately beneath the jaw or suprasternal

Thyroglossal
- Superficial unilocular cyst attached to hyoid bone and which moves upwards when tongue is protruded
- Refer for excision of cyst

Goitre
- Smooth midline swelling usually in adolescent girls. May be hyperthyroidism, but usually benign. Iodine deficiency rarely seen in UK.

RECURRENT ABDOMINAL PAIN

- Affects up to 10% of all children
- Often a strong family history of recurrent abdominal pain or headache

History
- Differentiate from organic causes by:

Table 4.1

Organic pathology	No organic pathology
Other symptoms, e.g. diarrhoea, vomiting, poor appetite	Healthy, normal appetite and growth
Pain peripheral	Pain central
No precipitating stress	Evidence of stress
No emotional disturbance	Other emotional disturbance
No secondary gain	Secondary gain, e.g. kept off school

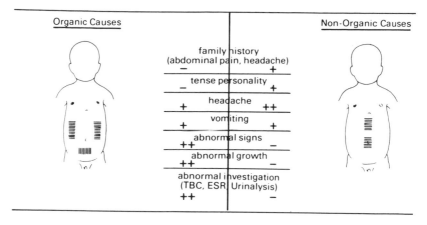

Organic Causes   Non-Organic Causes

	family history (abdominal pain, headache)	
−		+
	tense personality	
−		+
	headache	
+		++
	vomiting	
+		+
	abnormal signs	
++		−
	abnormal growth	
++		−
	abnormal investigation (TBC, ESR Urinalysis)	
++		−

Fig. 4.8 Features pointing to an organic cause of recurrent abdominal pain.

Examination
* Thorough examination to exclude abnormal physical signs helps to reassure parents and child
* Height and weight to confirm normal growth

Investigation
* Usually unnecessary; a battery of tests is costly and the act of investigation can cast parental doubts on the absence of physical illness
* In selected cases, if there is clinical doubt, urinalysis, full blood count, ESR and abdominal ultrasound should be undertaken

Management
* Reassure that there is no physical illness through careful physical examination, minimal investigation and explanation of how these exclude a physical cause
* Accept that the child is feeling real pain, but that the cause is 'muscle tension'. Explanations can follow the line: 'You know how the skin outside the body can change colour, go pale or blush, in response to how you feel, organs inside the body can do just the same, for example when you feel *butterflies* or if you go to the toilet a lot when you are worried'
* Child can receive comfort and understanding, but must go to school, attend lessons and should not be offered any medicines
* Offer follow-up if parents do not seem reassured
* Explanations often need to be repeated before they are understood and accepted
* Continued sympathetic support goes a long way

HEADACHES

Acute headache
- Most present as a feature of systemic febrile illness
  - Suspect meningitis/encephalitis if there is significant drowsiness, irritability, photophobia or focal neurological signs. Look for a purpuric rash (meningococcal)
  - It is also important to exclude a history of recent head injury with the above presenting signs. Both these groups need urgent referral

Recurrent headaches
- These are extremely common with an increasing incidence with age. 85% of boys and 93% of girls in secondary school report recurrent headaches. The vast majority of these have no obvious organic pathology, though can cause significant impairment to educational progress through absenteeism. 3–5% of all secondary school children suffer with migraine

Migraine
- Headache with vomiting, prostration and often strong family history (features of classical migraine)
- Visual symptoms (blurring, flashing lights or field defects) may accompany the other symptoms
- Features are often not classical
- Look for precipitating factors, i.e. hunger, fatigue, stress or foods (chocolate, cheese and caffeine)

Important points
- Diagnosis of exclusion with no focal neurological signs
- Residual neurological signs following an episode of headache (i.e. hemiplegic migraine) is a recognised complication of migraine though this is only transient and should resolve completely. Refer if in doubt

Management
- Full history plus examination
- Explanation of problem to child and parent
- Look for precipitating factors. May be useful to keep a diary to identify precipitants

Treatment
- Paracetamol plus rest given in early phase of headache
- Combined analgesic and anti-emetic (i.e. Migraleve) if the above fails
- Prophylactic treatment for recurrent migraine (i.e. greater than one time per week). Can use pizotifen or propranolol (contraindicated in asthmatics)

Anxiety or fatigue
* These are recognised causes of headache though stress management is sometimes difficult. Try to exclude bullying and encourage exercise which is known to alleviate stress to an extent. If exercise is suggested it should be on a regular basis

Sinusitis
* This may be clear from the history and associated with recurrent rhinorrhoea or tenderness over the sinuses. An X-ray of the sinuses will help identify the problem and responds to short courses of antibiotics if infective or antihistamines/decongestants if allergic

Ocular causes
* Hypermetropia and astigmatism may rarely cause headaches, though ocular causes are usually not significant precipitants of regular headaches. Consider referral to optician

Intracranial lesions
* This is the major differential diagnosis which warrants urgent referral. Suspect this if:
    — Headache wakes the child (as opposed to the child already awake and discovering he/she has a headache)
    — Recurrent morning headache
    — Increasing severity
    — Slowing of growth
    — Neurological signs

Assessment of children
* History, encompassing the above points
* Examination
    — Full neurological examination
    — Measurement of growth
    — Measurement of visual acuity
    — Measurement of blood pressure
    — Exclude obvious dental problems

PAINS IN THE LEGS

Causes

Trauma
* History important
* Look for greenstick fractures and soft-tissue injury
* Consider child abuse

Cramp
* Typical history, i.e. at rest
* May be helped by quinine (tonic water)

- Vitamin D deficiency should be excluded
- Cramp with exercise relieved by rest, consider muscle disorders, e.g. metabolic myopathies

Rickets
- Pain is often the presenting feature in adolescents
- Raised alkaline phosphatase

Joint disease
- Hip, knee and ankle movements should be examined in all cases
- Restricted movement, particularly in the hip, may indicate important disease such as slipped upper femoral epiphysis
- In all cases where there is pain and restricted movement or fixed deformity, X-ray is needed
- If there is increased movement past neutral, consider hypermobility syndrome

Osgood–Schlatter's disease
- Tender over tibial apophysis
- Common in adolescents
- Usually responds to rest
- Other osteochondritides affecting knee and ankle must also be considered

Rare though important causes
- Osteomyelitis
- Juvenile arthritis
- Leukaemia and tumours of bone

No cause found
- Many cases fit into this category
- Pain is often localized to insertion of tendons or the junction of the epiphysis and metaphysis
- Advise that a further appointment is needed if the pain gets worse or does not improve as some important conditions may have few physical signs early on
- In some children recurrent limb pains may be due to emotional disturbance, bullying

NON-ATTENDANCE AT SCHOOL – SCHOOL REFUSAL AND TRUANCY

- 80–90% of absence from school is due to illness
- 1% is due to school refusal
- Remainder is due to truancy and active withholding of the child from school
- 20% of 15 year olds may be truanting from school
- Truancy rates are included in school 'league tables'

Comparison of school refusal and truancy

Table 4.2 Comparison of school refusal and truancy

School refusal	Truancy
Small family	Large family
Social classes I, II, III	Social classes IV, V
Boys = girls	Boys > girls
Good school work	Poor school work
Used to enjoy school	Disliked school
Better prognosis	Poorer prognosis
Anxious, phobic	Antisocial
Fewer separations	More separations
Parental over-protection	Disinterested parents
Anxious parents	Inconsistent discipline + corporal punishment
Fathers not strongly supportive	History of absence of fathers

Management
- Exclude a physical illness by history and examination
  - Task may be difficult as:
  - Children with school phobia present with physical symptoms when under pressure and are better when not in school
  - Psychosomatic symptoms such as headache, abdominal pain may show clear temporal relationship to school attendance
  - For children who are being withheld or are truanting, physical illness may be presented as the cause. The child may indeed have a chronic physical illness such as asthma, but this is used as a smokescreen. Non-attendance may also result through undertreatment or poor compliance or where there is excessive parental anxiety about perceived additional health risks of sending their child to school
  - Genuine and forged or altered medical certificates may be presented

Truancy
- The Education Welfare Officer should be taking a leading role
- The paediatrician should consider history:
  - How long has child been truanting?
  - Has truanting occurred in a group or alone?
  - If not alone, who are the other pupils involved?
  - What is the family attitude towards truancy?
  - Are they punitive, disinterested or supportive of non-attendance?
  - What other concerns are there about health, conduct or care?
- An interview or a series of interviews with the child on his own will establish rapport and identify pressures that have led to truancy
- Deal with medical factors which might be contributing towards learning difficulties and liaise with the school over changes in teaching that might make the curriculum more relevant to the

child's needs and give success and satisfaction. Sometimes a change of school is requested and, where carefully thought through, can provide benefit

- Consider emotional or sexual abuse as possible underlying causes
- Consider drug or solvent abuse
- Recognise the risk that children who are truanting and not at home take of juvenile offending or exploitation by adults
- Greater parental involvement in supervising journey to and from school
- Encouraging regular liaison between parents and school, increasing their interest in and knowledge about what the child is doing
- Increase support given by pastoral care systems inside and outside school
- If these actions are not successful, prosecution may take place under the 1989 Children Act and an Educational Attendance Order obtained
- In some cases psychiatric referral may be appropriate, especially where there is evidence of distress, unusual behaviour or depression

School refusal
- Try to identify specific causes
  — Anxiety about separation
  — Collusion of parent
  — Anxiety about journey to school
  — Worries about individual lessons or teachers
  — Difficulties in relationships with peers
  — Anxiety about school dinners
  — Anxiety about using school lavatories
  — Worry about changing for games
- See regularly and discuss identified fears with child, parents, and school staff
- Provide sympathetic support, while at the same time insisting that the child must attend school
- A daily firm escort to school is often needed
- Key to success is an early return to school
- More resistant non-attendance may be dealt with by admission to special units such as tutorial classes or in-patient child psychiatric services for deeply established patterns of school refusal

BULLYING

Definition
- Bullying is the intentional, unprovoked abuse of power by one or more children inflicting pain or causing distress to another child on repeated occasions
- It is not bullying when two children of approximately the same physical or psychological strength fight or quarrel

Types of bullying
- Physical bullying
- Verbal bullying
- Gesture bullying
- Extortion bullying
- Exclusion bullying
- Sexual and racial harassment are particularly disturbing forms of verbal bullying

Myths about bullying
- Bullying doesn't harm anyone
- It is character-building
- It is a part of growing up

Epidemiology of bullying
- About one child in three is involved in bully/victim problems at some stage
- Approximately 10% are regularly bullied; 4% are severe bullies
- Most bullying happens in the same class and year group
- Boys tend to be bullied more physically, while girls suffer from more indirect forms of bullying
- Both bullies and victims tend to have poor curriculum attainment and are less popular with teaching staff
- Bullying takes place at school in playgrounds, corridors and dining rooms
- It also occurs in youth clubs, streets and on the way to and from school
- Bullying is not directly related to the size of the school or average class size
- It's higher in areas of social deprivation
- More than half the victims do not tell their teachers or parents about being bullied

Some characteristics of bullies and victims
Victims
- Passive, lacking in self-confidence
- Low self-esteem
- Physically weaker
- More likely to be 'different' (e.g. obese, disabled, different skin or hair colour, non-local accents)
- 'Provocative victims' may be hyperactive, seek out aggressive situations

Bullies
- Aggressive towards peers, parents, teachers
- Violent, disruptive, physically stronger
- Impulsive, lack self-control
- Involved in other forms of anti-social behaviour
- 'Anxious bullies' lack self confidence

Effects of bullying

Victims
- Loss of confidence and self-esteem
- Become withdrawn and unable to concentrate
- Poor academic performance
- School phobia
- Attempt suicide or self-harm
- In the long term adult victims of bullying may suffer:
  — Depression
  — Agoraphobia
  — Psychosomatic illnesses
  — Difficulties forming relationships
    ('love-shy')

Bullies
- Bullies are three times as likely to have a criminal conviction as the general population by the age of 24 and four times as likely to be multiple offenders

Warning signs of a child being bullied
- Unexplained injuries
- Non-specific physical complaints
- School refusal
- Changes in behaviour
- Attempted self-harm

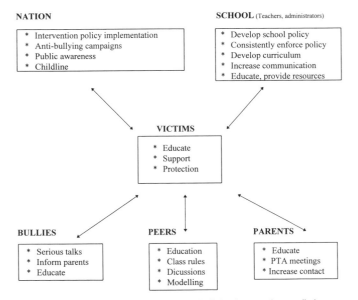

Fig. 4.9 Bullying. Modified from 'A school-based anti-bullying intervention: preliminary evaluation' by Debra Pepler et al from *Understanding and Managing Bullying*, edited by Delwyn Tattum, published by Heinemann, 1993.

Prevention
- National intervention programme
- Whole-school approach – good supervision, specific policy on bullying and general ethos
- At class level – clear rules and sanctions, groups work talks with individual victims, bullies and parents

Outcomes of intervention programmes
- 50% reduction in bully/victim problems
- Reduction in general anti-social behaviour
- Drop in truancy rates and increased pupil satisfaction and enjoyment of school life

BOWEL AND BLADDER CONTROL

Normal acquisition of bladder and bowel control
Natural history
- Most children attain daytime bowel and bladder control between the ages of 2 and 2.5 years
- Night time bladder control is attained by 90% at 5 years, and 95% at 10 years
- Up to 1% of adults continue to wet the bed

Acquisition of control may be hindered by:
- Medical problems
  - Structural
  - Neurological
  - Infective
- Learning difficulties
- Emotional problems
- Abuse and neglect
- Social problems
  - Chaos
  - Absence of training
- Familial patterns

Toilet training
- May be carried out from the age of 2 years if the child is developmentally ready, i.e.
  - Able to understand the task
  - Able to communicate his needs
  - Has appropriate gross and fine motor skills
  - Has a stable environment in which to carry out training
- This view is being challenged by those who point out that the move to later toilet training has been associated with an increase in continence problems; they would recommend:
  - An upper limit of 20 months to commence training

— For the child to sit on the pot as soon as able to sit stably
— Provided that this is done within a stable environment, and with an atmosphere that is relaxed and non-censorious, it is difficult to see how this can be harmful

Methods
- Imitation and demonstration:
  — Children learn most things from copying others
  — An older sibling may be the best instructor
- Regular 'potting' after meals with praise for success
- Formal behavioural programmes
- 'Exotic' such as the use of musical potties

Wetting in school children

Causes of nocturnal enuresis and daytime wetting
- 'Late maturation'
  — Most children with enuresis have no pathology but represent the tail end of a normal distribution
- Urinary tract infections
  — Up to 5% may have UTI
  — May be associated with anatomical abnormalities
- General developmental delay
- Neurological problems affecting bladder innervation
- Metabolic problems affecting urine volume or concentration
  — Diabetes mellitus or insipidus
- Family discord
  — At time of initial toilet training
  — Continued instability
- Sexual abuse

Wetting in older children

History
- When? Day/night?
- Primary or secondary?
- How often? Nights per week, days per week, times per night or day
- Any obvious pattern or course – e.g. too busy playing, late night, not in school holidays or at weekends, onset followed move, birth of sibling or bereavement?
- What is the child's bed-time?
- What is the interval between bed-time and wetting?
  — Does he wet shortly after going to bed and perhaps more than once a night or just once after 7–8 hours?
- What do the parents do if the child is wet?
- What does the child wear in bed?
  — Nappies or ordinary nightwear?
- Own bedroom? Own bed? Where is toilet?
- Is there any daytime frequency/urgency? (common)
- Is there a family history of bladder or bowel control problems?

- Are there any other medical, developmental or social problems?

Examination

In the absence of organic disease, treatment is usually not indicated before 6 years of age.

- Exclude organic cause by:
  - Urinalysis
  - General examination
  - BP
  - Neurological, (bladder S1 root), lower limb neurology, spine, reflexes
  - Height and weight
  - Radiology not necessary as a routine

Management (principles)

- Offer regular appointments (weekly for some younger children)
- Record kept by child and parent
- Praise for appropriate behaviour and support of parents to discourage criticism or intolerance
- Explanation to the child of anatomy and physiology (pictures of urine flow and bladder filling)
- Explanation to the child of brain's control over bladder (a muscle that can be trained)
- Explanation to the child about sleep (when we are asleep, many parts of the body carry on working as usual and others can be taught, e.g. you could probably wake up early if there was something exciting to do and sleep longer if there is no school)
- Stress personal responsibility of the child and recognise factors that might reward wetting, e.g. sleeping in parents' bed

Management (methods)

Charts

- Star for dry nights (or variations, e.g. colour in a picture)
  - Ignore wet nights
- Very effective and method of choice with young children
- Needs effective parental encouragement and regular appointments
- Must be combined with explanations as above

Alarms

- 80% become dry in 4 months
- 10% relapse but usually respond to a further trial
- The alarm is kept until the child is totally dry for at least 6 weeks
- Child
  - 7 years old or over (developmentally)
  - Own bed and bedroom desirable
  - Be motivated as nights are disturbed
- Teaching and 'rehearsal' are vital
  - Set up alarm with child and parent
  - Trigger alarm with saline

- Maintenance of equipment and correct techniques of use are vital; check for:
  — Low batteries
  — Loose connections
  — Alarm too near the bed so that the child can easily switch it off
- An alarm with a vibrator is available for deaf children; it can also be very useful for children who share a bedroom
- An alarm is now available for children with daytime wetting; it is worn rather like a *walkman*

Desmopressin
- Not as effective as the alarm
- Administered as nasal spray or tablets
- High relapse rate in some studies, but prolonged therapy is effective and safe
- May be useful for short-term use, e.g. on holiday
- Method of choice in children who are unsuccessful with alarms

Interval training
- This is recommended on the evidence that children with enuresis pass smaller volumes of urine at each voiding than children who are dry
  — They therefore have frequency of micturition if the fluid input is normal
  — Measures, therefore, that will increase daytime functional bladder capacity will also lead to improved function during sleep
  — The attached figure shows a system for interval training with a constant fluid input, but increasing intervals between micturition
  — Interval training is successful in about 50% of children, particularly those with urgency and frequency that is not caused by organic pathology
- The system is explained to the child by means of simple anatomical diagrams
- Getting through the night can be likened to learning to swim across a pool:
  — As you try harder you get further and further across, until you can do a whole width (i.e. wetting later and later in the night until you eventually get through to the next morning)
  — In the end, what is originally very difficult becomes easy
- When the child learns to fill the bladder up fully, this will wake him up, whereas a partly full bladder will not

Ten times routine

- Rehearsal ten times of getting out of bed and going to the toilet can lead to the child waking where needed
- Can be reinforced by leaving a 'calling card' in the toilet

Table 4.3 Bladder training regime

An alarm clock is useful to let you know when to have a drink or to go to the toilet. The drink can be anything that you like. If you cannot manage any particular day, the programme should be repeated the next day. By following the programme you will learn to carry more and more water for longer and longer. You must first learn to do this when you are awake and will then find staying dry at night much easier. Remember the bladder is a muscle and all muscles work better with training.

Day 1		Day 2		Day 3		Day 4		Day 5		Remarks
Take a drink every hour (about ½ pint)		Take a drink every hour (about ½ pint)		Take a drink every hour (about ½ pint)		Take a drink every hour (about ½ pint)		Take a drink every hour (about ½ pint)		
Go to toilet every 1 hour		Go to toilet every 1½ hours		Go to toilet every 2 hours		Go to toilet every 2½ hours		Go to toilet every 3 hours		
Drinks	*Toilet*	*Drinks*	*Toilet*	*Drinks*	*Toilet*	*Drinks*	*Toilet*	*Drinks*	*Toilet*	
9.00 a.m.	9.00 a.m.	9.00 a.m.	9.00 a.m.	9.00 a.m.	9.00 a.m.	9.00 a.m.	9.00 a.m.	9.00 a.m.	9.00 a.m.	
10.00 a.m.	10.00 a.m.	10.00 a.m.		10.00 a.m.		10.00 a.m.		10.00 a.m.		
11.00 a.m.	11.00 a.m.	11.00 a.m.	10.30 a.m.	11.00 a.m.	11.00 a.m.	11.00 a.m.		11.00 a.m.		
12.00 p.m.	12.00 p.m.	12.00 p.m.	12.00 p.m.	12.00 p.m.		12.00 p.m.	11.30 a.m.	12.00 p.m.	12.00 p.m.	
1.00 p.m.	1.00 p.m.	1.00 p.m.		1.00 p.m.	1.00 p.m.	1.00 p.m.		1.00 p.m.		
2.00 p.m.	2.00 p.m.	2.00 p.m.	1.30 p.m.	2.00 p.m.		2.00 p.m.	2.00 p.m.	2.00 p.m.	3.00 p.m.	
3.00 p.m.		2.00 p.m.	3.00 p.m.		3.00 p.m.	3.00 p.m.	4.30 p.m.	3.00 p.m.		

Imipramine

- Up to 30% cure rate has been claimed, but bearing in mind the high relapse rate, long-term success is probably achieved in only 10% if used alone
- Most useful if combined with other methods, e.g. charts
- Maximum effect in first week of use
- Dangers of accidental poisoning
- Try for 4–6 weeks in a dose of 25 mg (up to 75 mg can be given to secondary school children)
- Explanations are important: 'like a walking stick – it will help you to do better only if you try yourself'
- Can be useful for short-term use, e.g. on holiday
- Really only for third-line treatment if alarm, desmopressin and training programmes unsuccessful

SOILING

Causes
- Faulty training
    — Punitive or against a background of family stress
- Absent training
- Continuing response to stress
- Constipation with overflow
- Abuse or neglect

In encopresis the stools are passed in inappropriate places or hidden.

Management
- Exclude organic causes:
    — Learning difficulties
    — Chronic constipation
- Explanation of problem to child and parents
- Introduce record and reward system for passing stools appropriately
    — A 'pooh' chart in which the child draws what he has passed is popular and successful with young children
- A step under the child's feet to relax the perineum while seated on the toilet
- Measures such as a story tape or picture books kept in the toilet
- Introduce a training programme of toileting after meals
    — This can be combined with a pleasant activity such as being read a story
- Laxatives if there is constipation:
    — Dioctyl sodium sulphosuccinate is useful to soften stools where they have become painful to pass or where there are (or have been) painful peri-anal lesions such as a fissure
    — A stimulant laxative, e.g. senokot is often needed in addition
    — Sodium picosulphate is useful if senokot proves ineffective

- Rarely, if constipation is gross, it is necessary to commence treatment with a microlax enema or glycerin suppository
- Anal dilatation under general anaesthesia may also be tried in persistent cases
• Stress personal responsibility of the child
• Modify the parental response and support parents
- Sometimes the child is not the patient
• Most will need support and supervision for 1–2 years
• Psychiatric referral or in-patient treatment is required where the above measures prove inadequate

SLEEP

• Sleep problems are common in childhood and are one of the commonest reasons for consultation with the community paediatrician
• Prevalence
- Difficulty falling asleep: 22% of 9 month olds, 15–20% of toddlers, and 16% of 3 year olds
- Frequent waking in the night: 42% of 9 month olds, 20–26% of toddlers, and 14% of 3 year olds. Half the frequent wakers will have settling problems
• The emotional and physical strain which sleep problems cause for the rest of the family can be considerable; arguments, irritability, poor work performance, curtailment of sexual and social life
• Persistent sleep difficulties may lead to violence inflicted upon a partner or child and because of this need to be taken seriously and prevented where possible

Types of problem

Amount of sleep
• Particularly when this does not match parental expectations
• Many normal newborn babies have sleep/wake cycles of about 4 hours determined by hunger
• By 12 weeks most have moved to a diurnal cycle and 70% are reported to sleep through the night
• Older children may need only 8–10 hours sleep and yet be expected to sleep 12–14 hours

Night waking
• All children (and adults) wake briefly in the night and settle back to sleep
• Common but improves with maturity:
- 20% of 1–2 year olds wake five or more nights a week
- 14% of 3 year olds wake three or more nights a week
- 3% of 8 year olds wake three or more nights a week

- However, there is high continuity:
  - Half of all-night-waking 1 year olds will continue to do so 6 months later
  - A third of night-waking 3 year olds will continue to do so 1 year later

Settling difficulties
- More persistent:
  - 16% of 3 year olds
  - 15% of 4 year olds
  - 10% of 8 year olds

Early morning waking
- Most troublesome in the 18–36 month age group
- Effect will depend upon parental lifestyle
- A combination of night waking, settling difficulties and early morning waking is common

Dreams and nightmares
- Occur during light (rapid eye movement) sleep
- Common in 3–4 year olds
- Not usually associated with emotional problems
- May be due to overheating

Night terrors
- Occur mainly in children over 5
- The child screams out, is often sweating and appears terrified, but is difficult to wake and has no memory of the event the next day
- Occurs in stage 4 (deep) sleep, unassociated with emotional problems
- Parents need reassurance about the normality and self-limiting nature of these happenings

Sleep walking
- Also a stage 4 phenomenon of older children

General approach to evaluation of sleep problems
- Assess the extent of the problem
- Exclude medical causes where possible by careful history taking and physical examination
- Assess any additional social and environmental risk factors
- Treatment programmes
  - Behaviour management
  - Medication
  - Psychotherapy
- Extent of the problem
  - When did it start, the type and pattern of disturbance, the effect on the family, parental expectations, parental responses, ploys already tried
- Exclusion of medical causes. Consider:
  - Chronic illness

Asthma – nights disturbed by coughing/distress
Obstructive sleep apnoea – snoring, recurrent URTIs,
rhinitis and hayfever
Chronic serous otitis – pain and discomfort
— Prematurity – not uncommon for babies to have been ill in
the newborn period and isolated from mother leading to later
parental separation anxieties
— Difficulties in first and second years usually settle by the
third
— Special needs – children with significant learning disabilities
may have problems in attaining normal sleep stages and
diurnal pattern as a result of CNS damage. Parents may
be overresponsive to the child and reinforce the sleep
difficulties
— Temperament – some children have a low sensory threshold

Assessment of social and environmental factors
• Consider maternal absences, depression, illness or accidents,
marital difficulties, alcohol or drug abuse; all factors which may
contribute to the difficulties
• Are there problems with the adequacy of the housing: noise,
dampness, poor heating, excess light?
• Breast-fed babies tend to be more wakeful than bottle fed –
expectation to be picked up and cuddled. There is no evidence that
earlier introduction of solids to the diet makes a difference
• In some cultures it is common for the baby to sleep in the parental
bed and there is no evidence that this practice is associated with an
increased prevalence of wakefulness

Management
Simple measures suitable for a first consultation
• *During the day* ensure that the child has:
— Exercise
— Fresh air
— Regular play time
— Regular meals
— Time with mother
• *At bed time* a familiar routine (cueing technique), e.g.:
— Bath
— Warm drink (clean teeth)
— Own bed (adequate bedding)
— Own room (where possible)
— Quiet play time (story or look at picture book)
— Cuddly toy or security blanket
— Lighting (night light, effective curtains)
• *During the night:*
— Respond consistently
— Avoid anger

— More effective to go after 5–10 minutes and quietly comfort, than to go immediately and in anger

More structured behavioural techniques

- Parents given a chart (sleep diary) to record sleep pattern
- Initially weekly appointments until recordings improve, then fortnightly or monthly
  — Support of parents is just as important as specific advice on management

Treatment options

- Choice depends upon evaluation and parental preference

Relaxation techniques

- Consider light supper instead of milk to stop night hunger
- Bedtime routine as described
- Soothing and relaxing techniques to settle child, e.g. stroking, massage, rocking
- Relaxing sounds, e.g. lullaby, taped music, womb sound record or mechanical sounds such as ticking clock. (Another re-invention of the wheel!)
- For night waking, repeat relaxation technique with minimum stimulation, i.e. no change in lighting, no talking, no drinks
- If parent has to sit with the child they should be boring, e.g. take something to do

Extinction technique for well established behaviour

- If child comes into parents' bed (and this is not acceptable to them), the child is returned quietly to his own bed until the behaviour stops
- If the child cries, it is all right to go in every 5–10 minutes to check, but with minimal interaction between parent and child
- Extinction techniques are easy to recommend, sound in theory and very demanding in practice

Shaping technique

- Moving from unacceptable to desired pattern of behaviour in a gradual series of small steps, e.g. for a child who will not settle until 11 p.m., move the bedtime routine in a series of steps from 10.30 p.m. to 10 p.m. etc.

Positive reinforcement

- Only useful for children over 3 years of age
- Stickers or other rewards, e.g. a small present under the pillow, can be earned for desired behaviour, e.g. staying in own room, not going to parents until alarm rings
- In the case of the sleep-walking child safety issues are paramount and window latches and doors should be secured to prevent escape from the house!

For night terrors

- These usually occur at a fairly predictable time of night, matched to the level of the child's sleep

- Briefly waking the child, and then re-settling him or her immediately, just before this time is reached, is often very effective
- Waking the child when he appears restless will have the same effect

Drug treatment
- Not justified as a first line of action
- Useful in breaking the cycle of parental sleep deprivation leading to an inability to undertake behavioural approaches
- Usually for short-term use
- More effective for initiating sleep than for prolonging it or preventing night waking
- Dose must be adequate
  - Too little may have a reverse effect
- Should not be used as a short cut to avoid counselling
- Recommended medication: trimeprazine tartrate 3 mg/kg

Other
- There are a number of popular manuals and advice booklets for parents
- Parents may have access to a telephone helpline
- Early postnatal anticipation and guidance may prevent the establishment of long-term sleep difficulties in infants

THE CRYING BABY

- Crying is the baby's response to any negative feeling or experience
- Crying is a powerful stimulus for parental action – it may produce a comforting response, anger, exhaustion, confusion or feelings of inadequacy
- Its extent depends upon the nature and strength of the provoking event, the temperament of the baby, the response of the parent and the general characteristics of the physical and social environment
- It represents a need to be met: failure to respond in the young baby can result in apathy and withdrawal

Consider the following
- Is the character of the cry normal or abnormal?
  - If abnormal, investigate urgently, as serious illness or injury may be present
- Is the excessive crying of very recent onset and unusual for the child?
  - Indicates illness
- Is the crying associated with feeding?
  - May be due to too slow or too rapid delivery of milk, painful lesions in the mouth, nasal obstruction or may reflect mother's anxiety about feeding her baby
- Is the crying an established behaviour pattern?
  - If yes, may reflect stresses within the family, neglect or unhappiness (but may be more often quiet and withdrawn)

- Inappropriate handling unrelated to family stress may also lead to prolonged crying
- In some babies, despite good handling and a normal environment, a difficult temperament leads to prolonged crying
- The above causes need to be distinguished from normal episodic crying (short duration), in response to hunger, discomfort, boredom or anger

Management
- Exclude or treat organic disease by careful history and examination
  - This may need to be repeated, particularly in the prodromal stage of infectious diseases
  - Ascribing crying to 'wind' can be dangerous if it leads to serious problems being overlooked
  - If the baby is teething, as indicated by excessive salivation, fingers thrust into mouth, analgesics may help, but this diagnosis can also lead to serious problems being overlooked
  - Also look for signs of injury or neglect
- Obtain a detailed history of the pattern of crying through the day
  - Sympathetic listening is often therapeutic and can also identify causes
- Carrying and comforting the baby is the obvious thing to do, but many parents are confused about what is 'right'
  - As one mother commented, 'if a baby cries in a room of adults, half the adults will criticise her if she picks up the baby and the other half will criticise her if she does not'
  - Strongly support the need of the baby for comfort and the success of this simple approach but also acknowledge the conflict between the baby's demands, which might seem endless, and the parents' stamina, which might not match those demands
  - Simple measures, such as carrying the baby in a sling, sitting him up to see what is happening, a change of routine with more 'walks' outdoors, are often helpful
  - Give further advice on stimulation and appropriate responses: not anger; things to look at, listen to, play with, and company; look at how the day is structured; look at how the baby's needs are anticipated
- Assess the development of the child
  - Reassurance that development is normal will relieve a lot of parental worries
  - Is there general delay?
  - Are there any hearing, vision or (in the older child) speech problems?
  - Are there any other behaviour problems?
  - Are parental expectations realistic?

- Provide on-going support and a 'lifeline' for parents who are under stress, have no family support, are lone parents
- Consider admission to hospital if thought to be at risk or parents exhausted
- A day nursery or family centre place may also provide respite for a parent under stress, but must be combined with help for the underlying problem

IMMUNIZATION

Counselling
- Necessary to ensure that parents are making an informed decision
- Not giving an immunization is taking a greater risk than giving immunizations

UK recommended schedule

Birth
- BCG for high-risk children:
  — Asian or African (not Afrocaribbean)
  — History of TB in a relative living nearby
- Hepatitis B course:
  — For children of hepatitis B carriers, particularly if e-antigen-positive

Primary course

2 months
- 1st diphtheria/pertussis/tetanus, oral polio
- *Haemophilus influenzae* b (Hib)

3 months (4 weeks after first)
- 2nd diphtheria/pertussis/tetanus, oral polio
- *Haemophilus influenzae* b (Hib)

4 months (4 weeks after 2nd)
- 3rd diphtheria/pertussis/tetanus, oral polio
- *Haemophilus influenzae* b (Hib)

12–15 months
- Measles/mumps/rubella (MMR)

4–5 years (or 3 years after primary course)
- Diphtheria/tetanus, oral polio
- 2nd measles/mumps/rubella (MMR)

10–14 years
- BCG if tuberculin-negative
  — Rubella for girls not previously immunized (in the UK, this refers to girls born before 1988, who also missed the mass immunization campaign of school children in 1994)

15–19 years
- Tetanus, oral polio/low dose diphtheria

Recommended immunization schedule in the USA

2, 4 and 6 months
- Diphtheria/tetanus/pertussis + oral polio

1 year
- Measles/rubella or measles/mumps/rubella + tuberculin test

1.5 years
- Diphtheria/tetanus/pertussis + oral polio

4–6 years
- Diphtheria/tetanus/pertussis + oral polio

14–16 years
- Tetanus

- There are other satisfactory schedules used in other countries
- If a baby is born early, no allowance is made in the date for commencing immunization
  — Immunization starts 3 months from birth irrespective of prematurity

Upper age limits:
- Polio
  — None
  — Adults going to developing countries may need a booster or full course
- Diphtheria
  — Older children may have an adverse reaction
  — For children over 10 years use special adult (low-dose) vaccine or one-fifth dose of ordinary vaccine if the former is not available (0.1 ml)
  — A Schick test is not needed if adult vaccine is used
- Tetanus
  — None
  — Children and adults need a booster if they sustain a dirty cut and it is more than 10 years since the last injection
- Pertussis
  — A full course (three injections) is considered sufficient protection
  — Older children (beyond 6th birthday) may be immunized if there are younger children who they may pass the disease on to
- MMR – none
- Measles – it is rarely worthwhile immunizing adults
- BCG – none if tuberculin negative
- Rubella – none

General
- If longer gaps are left between doses they do not need to be repeated; it just means that full protection is delayed
- An immunization course never needs to be restarted

Contraindications and special considerations

General contraindications
- Acute illness especially with fever. Delay till fever settles
- Immunodeficiency states:
  - This includes oral steroid therapy but only if more than 2 mg/kg/day for more than a week is taken
  - Live vaccines should not be given in the following 3 months
  - For other conditions
    Live vaccines are contraindicated
    Discuss with specialist in charge
- Pregnancy:
  - Live vaccines should not be given, unless risk from the disease is very high

Specific
Pertussis
- Contraindications: severe local or general reaction to a preceding dose
  - Definition of a local reaction – an extensive area of redness and swelling which becomes indurated and involves most of the anterolateral surface of the thigh or a major part of the circumference of the upper arm
  - Definition of a general reaction: any of the following: fever >40.50°C, anaphylaxis, bronchospasm, laryngeal oedema, generalized collapse, prolonged unresponsiveness, convulsions occurring within 72 hours (and unexplained by any other cause)
- Special considerations
  - NOT contraindication, i.e. discuss with consultant in charge of case
  - Children with a documented history of cerebral damage in the neonatal period (good practice to include absence of a contraindication in the neonatal discharge summary)
  - Children with a personal history of convulsions

MMR
- Special considerations:
  - Severe egg allergy (anaphylaxis)
  - Neomycin and polymixin sensitivity (very rare in children)
  - If there is a personal or family history of febrile convulsions, MMR should be given after counselling the parents on the management of febrile reactions

Rubella
- Contraindications:
  - Pregnancy
- Special considerations:
  - Arthritis can be exacerbated

BCG
- Special considerations:
  - Grades III and IV Heaf
  - Positive reaction to tuberculin test should be followed by investigation, not immunization
  - No vaccine should be given if HIV-positive

Immunization myths
- History of allergic disease in the child or family is not a contraindication to any immunization nor are neurological conditions which are stable, e.g. cerebral palsy
- Snuffles or slight chestiness in a child who is otherwise well is not a reason for postponing any immunization
- A history of whooping cough or measles does not mean that you cannot immunize against these illnesses. The diagnosis is often uncertain and it is safer to immunize
- A child on antibiotics or any other medicine (except immunosuppressants) can be immunized if generally well
- Breast feeding and blood transfusions do not interfere with immunizations

Adverse reactions
Diphtheria/pertussis/tetanus
- Local redness and swelling, mild pyrexia and malaise, 1–2 days after injection

Pertussis
- Encephalopathy with serious or persisting problems 1 in 300 000 injections

Polio
- Paralytic polio 1–3 cases/million doses

MMR
Measles
- A mild measles-like illness 7–10 days after injection
- Febrile convulsions, though much less commonly than with naturally acquired measles

Mumps
- Parotid swelling in third week after immunization
- Meningoencephalitis rare (1/400 000)

Rubella
- Mild rubella-like illness
- Arthralgia (rare in children)

Anaphylaxis
- Can occur with any immunization, but is extremely rare
- Adrenaline must always be available (1/1 000)

— 0.05 ml	1 year old	⎫	i.m. repeated at
— 0.4 ml	4 year old	⎬	10 minutes and
— 0.5–0.75 ml	adult	⎭	30 minutes if necessary

Travel abroad

- Immunization against cholera, typhoid, polio and yellow fever may be recommended depending upon the country to be visited
- Yellow fever and cholera immunization are essential for entry into some countries
- Recommendations are reviewed annually and are published in *Health Advice for Travellers*, published by the Department of Health; telephone enquiries can also be made to the Hospital for Tropical Diseases Travel Clinic, tel: 0171 637 9899
- Malaria prophylaxis is also widely required, e.g. for Africa, Asia, South America
    - Asian families returning to India or Pakistan are at risk and require protection
    - Recommended antimalarials depend on the pattern of resistance in the country to be visited; advice may be obtained from the Malaria Reference Laboratory, tel: 0171 636 3924

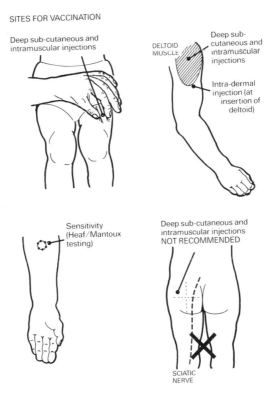

Fig. 4.10 Sites for vaccination.

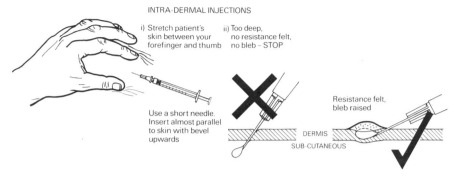

Fig. 4.11 Technique for intradermal injections.

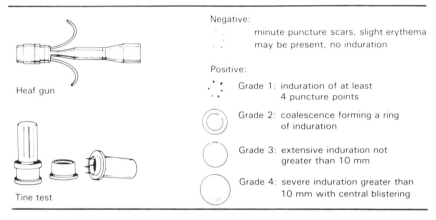

Heaf gun

Tine test

Negative:

minute puncture scars, slight erythema may be present, no induration

Positive:

Grade 1: induration of at least 4 puncture points

Grade 2: coalescence forming a ring of induration

Grade 3: extensive induration not greater than 10 mm

Grade 4: severe induration greater than 10 mm with central blistering

Fig. 4.12 The test is read after 72 hours. Children with negative reactions are given BCG; children with grade 1 reactions should also be given BCG unless previously immunized; children with a grade 2 reaction should be referred if no previous BCG has been given; all grade 3 and 4 reactions need X-ray and follow-up.

INFECTION

AIDS/HIV infection

- Organism – human immunodeficiency virus (HIV)

Clinical summary

- Spectrum of HIV infection from asymptomatic to AIDS

Vulnerable groups are:

- Homosexual/bisexual
- Intravenous drug abusers
- Via transfusion of blood or blood products that are untreated (all are now treated in UK)

- Children of affected mothers
- Female partners of men at risk

Children most likely to be infected by vertical transmission
- Pre-natal transmission occurs
- Probable transmission at birth due to exposure to maternal blood

People at risk:
- IV drug abusers
- Sexual partners of IV drug abusers
- Sexual partners of bisexual men
- Prostitutes
- Sexual partners of haemophiliacs
- Sexual partners of men in/from AIDS endemic areas

Presentations – adults:
- Pneumocystis carinii pneumonia
- Kaposi's sarcoma
- CNS infections e.g. *Toxoplasma*, Herpes Simplex, Papovavirus – may present with general symptoms or focal signs
- Alimentary, e.g. intractable diarrhoea, oesophageal candidiasis
- Pyrexia of unknown origin
- Lymphoma and other tumours
- Lymphadenopathy associated with other illness, e.g. candida, shingles, impetigo, weight loss, diarrhoea

Presentations – children:
- Recurrent bacterial infections
- Failure to thrive
- Severe/persistent oral thrush
- Recurrent diarrhoea
- Generalized lymphadenopathy
- Hepatosplenomegaly
- Progressive encephalopathy
- Loss of developmental milestones

Incubation period
- Anti-HIV antibodies detectable 3–12 weeks after exposure

Infectious period
- All antigen-positive individuals must be regarded as being able to transmit the infection

Method of spread
- Sexual intercourse
- Untreated blood and blood products
- Shared needles
- It cannot be acquired from food or shared utensils, toilets, swimming pools, kissing, musical instruments, or any other casual contact
- Apart from transfusion and vertical transmission, infectivity is low – less than for hepatitis B

Exclusion period
- None
- Normal social contact between children carries no risk

Diagnosis
- HIV antibody test
  - A negative test, except in very early infection, excludes AIDS
  - A positive test does not mean that the patient will develop the disease, but is at individual risk and can transmit it to others
  - Diagnosis is difficult under 15 months due to persistence of maternal antibodies

Campylobacter gastroenteritis
- Organism – *Campylobacter* species

Clinical summary
- Diarrhoea, blood in stool, abdominal pain, systemic upset, prostration, vomiting in children

Incubation period
- Commonly 2–4 days (extreme limits 1–10 days)

Infectious period
- Throughout illness unless an antibiotic is given

Method of spread
- Food, water
- Hand → mouth
- From pets (puppies and kittens)
- Moderately infectious

Exclusion period
- Until the child is clinically well

Diagnosis
- Microbiological

Management
- General measures for gastroenteritis
- Erythromycin, in severe infection, preferably given early

Chicken pox
- Organism – Herpes virus – Varicella/Zoster
- May be lethal in children with immunodeficiencies – they should be given specific immunoglobulin if in contact

Clinical summary
- Crops of vesicles most dense on the trunk

Incubation period
- Commonly 13–17 days (extreme limits 13–21 days)

Infectious period
- 1–2 days before rash appears, to 6 days after rash first appears

Method of spread
- Droplet or direct contact
- Highly infectious

Exclusion period
- Until 6 days after the appearance of the rash

Diagnosis
- Clinical

Management
- Conservative
- Analgesics and antipruritics

Cholera

- Organism – *Vibrio cholerae*
- Vaccine available, e.g. foreign travel
- Notifiable in UK

Clinical summary
- Profuse watery diarrhoea followed by vomiting, shock and collapse
- Can be mild or asymptomatic
- Within 1 week of return from an endemic country or contact with a carrier

Incubation period
- Commonly 2–3 days (extreme limits few hours to 5 days)

Infectious period
- Variable – until stools are negative
- There are carriers

Method of spread
- Contaminated food or water
- Highly infectious

Exclusion period
- Seek expert advice

Diagnosis
- Clinical + microbiological

Management
- Oral or intravenous rehydration
- Antibiotic to eradicate *Vibrio* from gastrointestinal tract (<10 years cotrimoxazole, >10 years tetracycline)

Common cold

- Organism – Rhinoviruses, Adenoviruses

Clinical summary
- Coryza

Incubation period
- 1–5 days

Infectious period
- Average 6–7 days

Method of spread
- Droplet
- Infectivity high

Exclusion period
- As indicated by clinical condition, unless in contact with high risk patients

Diagnosis
- Clinical

Management
- Symptomatic

Croup

- Organism – Para-influenza, influenza, respiratory syncytial viruses

Clinical summary
- Barking cough, hoarse voice and stridor

Incubation period
- Few days to 1 week

Infectious period
- While symptoms persist

Method of spread
- Droplet

Exclusion period
- Until asymptomatic

Diagnosis
- Clinical – *do not use tongue depressor to examine throat*

Management
- Supportive, humidified air

Diphtheria

- Organism – *Corynebacterium diphtheriae*
- Notifiable in UK
- Vaccine available – routine immunization

Clinical summary
- Severe prostration

- Adherent greyish membrane/exudate causing upper respiratory tract obstruction
- Complications due to exotoxin include myocarditis and paralysis

Incubation period
- Commonly 2–5 days (extreme limits 2–7 days)

Infectious period
- Variable – usually 2–4 weeks from first signs
- There are carriers

Method of spread
- Droplet or direct contact
- Moderately infectious

Exclusion period
- Seek expert advice

Diagnosis
- Clinical
- Microbiological confirmation takes 3–5 days

Management
- Erythromycin can be used to treat carriers
- Cases treated with antitoxin + erythromycin + general measures
- Must treat before microbiological confirmation available

Epiglottitis

- Organism – *Haemophilus influenzae*

Clinical summary
- Severe stridor of rapid onset, systemic illness, toxic

Incubation period
- Uncertain, 2–4 days?

Infectious period
- Until 24 hours of appropriate antibiotic treatment is complete

Method of spread
- Droplet

Exclusion period
- Until clinical recovery

Diagnosis
- Clinical – *do not use tongue depressor or examine throat*; radiology, bacteriology

Management
- Intravenous ampicillin
- Treat as emergency in hospital

Erythema infectiosum ('fifth disease'/'slapped cheek syndrome')

- Organism – Human Parvovirus B19

Clinical summary
- Mild illness of young children with characteristic erythema of cheeks (slapped face appearance)

Incubation period
- 7–22 days

Infectious period
- Unclear

Method of spread
- Droplet

Exclusion period
- Nil

Diagnosis
- Clinical

Management
- No specific measures indicated

Gastroenteritis

- See also under individual headings: *Campylobacter, Shigella, Giardia*
- Notifiable in the UK if due to food poisoning (any cause)

Clinical summary
- Vomiting, diarrhoea, abdominal pain
- Predominant symptom varies depending on cause, e.g.:

> *Rotavirus* – mainly diarrhoea
> *Staphylococcus* – vomiting

Cause
- These symptoms may also be due to a surgical or metabolic cause
- Often no causal organism found on routine stool culture
- Many cases are viral and can be found only by electron microscopy
- If many cases, suspect food poisoning
- Cases of food poisoning are notifiable
- Clusters of cases should be notified so that the source can be traced and further spread prevented

Microbiology

Bacterial:	*Viral:*	*Protozoal:*
Campylobacter	Rotavirus (50%)	*Giardia*
Shigella	Echovirus	*Cryptosporidium*
Escherichia coli	Coxsackie	
Salmonella	Adenovirus	

Table 4.4 Food poisoning

	Sources	Clinical	Incubation
Salmonella	Common in raw meat and may contaminate cooked or processed meat if not stored properly	Mainly diarrhoea	12–48 hours
Clostridium welchii	Cooked meat. Resistant to heating. Multiplies in anaerobic conditions	Abdominal pain Diarrhoea	12–48 hours
Staphylococcus	Meat Sweets Food handler is a carrier	Vomiting	30 mins–6 hours.
Bacillus Cereus	Fried rice kept warm	Vomiting	1–6 hours
Campylobacter	Poultry	Diarrhoea Abdominal pain Prolonged prostration	12–48 hours

Table 4.5 Clinical assessment of dehydration

Sign	5% dehydration	10% dehydration
Skin	Loss of turgor	Mottled, poor capillary return
Fontanelle	Depressed	Deeply depressed
Eyes	Sunken	Deeply sunken
Peripheral pulses	Normal	Tachycardia, poor volume
Mental state	Lethargic	Prostration, coma

Clostridium perfringens (former name: *Cl. welchii*)
Staphylococcus
Bacillus cereus

- Microbiological diagnosis may be very useful if there is a cluster of cases or a history of foreign travel
- If food poisoning is suspected, ensure that samples of food are kept for examination

Incubation period
- Varies widely depending upon organism, e.g.:

Staphylococcus	0.5 to 6 hours
Salmonella	12 to 48 hours
Cl. perfringens	12 to 48 hours
Rotavirus	48 hours
Campylobacter	3 to 5 days

Infectious period
- While organisms excreted in stools
- Cases due to toxins are not directly infectious, e.g. staphylococcal

Method of spread
- Faeces → hand → mouth
- Food → mouth

- Infectivity partly dependent upon hygiene, age of child, toilet training

Exclusion period
- Until acute diarrhoea has stopped

Diagnosis
- Usually clinical in community practice

Management
- Stop solid foods
- Glucose/electrolyte solution in frequent small amounts for 24–48 hours with gradual return to normal diet after that
- If dehydration over 5%, admit
- Stress importance of general hygiene in preventing spread
- Involve public health department if food poisoning is suspected

Giardiasis

- Organism – protozoal – *Giardia lamblya*

Clinical summary
- Chronic diarrhoea

Incubation period
- 5–25 days

Infectious period
- During symptoms
- There are carriers, and infection may circulate within the family

Method of spread
- Faeces → hand → mouth
- Low infectivity

Exclusion period
- None

Diagnosis
- Cysts and adult form in stool
- Single negative result may be misleading

Management
- Metronidazole
- Look for infection in other family members

Glandular fever

- Organism – Epstein–Barr virus

Clinical summary
- Malaise, fever, sore throat, lymphadenopathy, rash, post-viral debility

Incubation period
- 4–6 weeks

Infectious period
- Prolonged beyond illness
- Sufferers are often infectious for a long time
- Since infectivity is low they are not a hazard in school
- Other family members are likely to catch the illness

Method of spread
- Very close contact
- Low infectivity

Exclusion period
- Nil for school children

Diagnosis
- Clinical + positive Paul Bunnell/Monospot (may not become positive for 3–4 weeks after onset of symptoms)

Management
- Symptomatic

Haemophilus infection

- Organism – *Haemophilus influenzae* – several serotypes
- Meningitis notifiable in UK
- Vaccine available – type b (type b usually responsible for *Haemophilus* meningitis in UK) – routine immunization

Clinical summary
- Meningitis, epiglottitis, septic arthritis, cellulitis, bacteraemia, pneumonia and empyema

Incubation period
- Uncertain – 2–4 days?

Infectious period
- As long as infection present or until 24 hours of antibiotic received

Method of spread
- Direct contact and droplet

Exclusion period
- Until clinically well

Diagnosis
- Clinical + bacteriological/immunological

Management
- General measures, depending on type of infection
- Antibiotics: meningitis – chloramphenicol or cefotaxime
  epiglottitis – chloramphenicol or cefotaxime
  arthritis – amoxycillin or cephuroxime
  contacts – rifampicin

Hand, foot and mouth disease

- Organism – Coxsackie A virus

Clinical summary
- Varies widely in severity
- Pyrexia, vesicles on hands and feet, and in mouth
- Difficulty feeding

Incubation period
- 3–5 days

Infectious period
- Acute phase of illness

Method of spread
- Direct contact; faecal → hand → mouth; droplet
- Infectivity low

Exclusion period
- During acute phase of illness

Diagnosis
- Clinical

Management
- Analgesics, fluids

Head lice/nits (pediculosis capitis)

- Organism – *Pediculus humanus* (var. *capitis*)

Clinical summary
- Eggs (nits) or adult lice seen in hair

Incubation period
- 7 days

Infectious period
- As long as living (untreated) lice remain in the hair

Method of spread
- Very close contact
- Infectivity low

Exclusion period
- Until treatment started

Diagnosis
- Clinical

Management
- Malathion, carbaryl, permethrin, phenothrin
- Lotion preferable to shampoo (contact with hair generally too short), aqueous preparations preferable to alcoholic (can exacerbate asthma)

- The hair is shampooed and combed after 12 hours
- Check other family members and treat if affected
- Rotate treatments according to local policy to reduce problems of resistance

Hepatitis A (infectious hepatitis)

- Organism – Hepatitis A virus
- Notifiable in the UK
- Vaccine available, e.g. foreign travel

Clinical summary
- Jaundice, fever, malaise, enlarged liver
- Infection may be very mild in young children who are often not clinically jaundiced

Incubation period
- Commonly 28–30 days (extreme limits 15–50 days)

Infectious period
- 14 days before jaundice to 7 days after

Method of spread
- Direct contact; faecal → oral; contaminated food or water
- Moderately infectious

Exclusion period
- 7 days from jaundice starting

Diagnosis
- Clinical
- Liver function tests + antigen

Management
- General supportive measures

Hepatitis B (serum hepatitis)

- Organism – Hepatitis B virus
- Notifiable in the UK
- Vaccine available, e.g.:
  — Close family contacts of a case or carrier
  — Infants born to mothers who have had hepatitis B, or who are carriers
  — Those receiving regular transfusions of blood or blood products, and relatives responsible for administration
  — Patients with chronic renal failure
  — High-risk occupations

Clinical summary
- Jaundice, fever, malaise, enlarged liver

Incubation period
- Commonly 28–30 days (extreme range 15–50 days)

Infectious period
- Infectious before and during illness
- There are carriers

Method of spread
- Sexual intercourse
- Nursing mother to child
- Untreated blood and blood products
- Shared needles
- Infectivity low

Exclusion period
- Nil once well

Diagnosis
- Clinical
- Liver function tests + detection of antigen

Management
- Supportive + treatment of complications, which are common giving hepatitis B a poorer prognosis

Herpes simplex

- Organism – Herpes virus type 1

Clinical summary
- Important in immunodeficient children
- Primary infection more widespread and serious than secondary (recurrent) lesions
- May produce gingivostomatitis, cold sores, keratoconjunctivitis, encephalitis

Incubation period
- 2–12 days

Infectious period
- Variable, can be several weeks
- There are carriers

Method of spread
- Close contact
- Low infectivity

Exclusion period
- Nil

Diagnosis
- Usually clinical

Management
- Acyclovir, given as early as possible

Impetigo

- Organism – *Staphylococcus, Streptococcus* species

Clinical summary
- Multiple vesicles with golden yellow crusts

Incubation period
- *Streptococcus*: 1–3 days
- *Staphylococcus*: 4–10 days

Infectious period
- While lesions are present

Method of spread
- Direct contact
- Infectivity high

Exclusion period
- Until lesions have healed

Diagnosis
- Clinical + microbiology

Management
- Topical fusidic acid or mupirocin
- Oral erythromycin or flucloxacillin for more severe or extensive lesions

Influenza

- Organism – Influenza viruses
- Vaccine available, e.g. patients with severe chronic respiratory or cardiac disease

Clinical summary
- Pyrexia, malaise, headache, cough, myalgia
- Complications: pneumonia, otitis media

Incubation period
- 2–3 days

Infectious period
- The 3 days before onset of symptoms

Exclusion period
- Until clinically well

Method of spread
- Droplet spread
- Infectivity high

Diagnosis
- Clinical

Management
- General measures

Malaria

- Organism – protozoal – *Plasmodium* species
- Notifiable in the UK
- Prophylaxis recommended for those visiting endemic areas

Clinical summary
- Cyclical fever, rigors, anaemia, splenomegaly
- History of travel to endemic areas

Incubation period
- 12–30 days, depending upon type (extreme range 8–10 months)

Infectious period
- Not infectious in UK (no vector)

Method of spread
- Mosquito bite in endemic areas
- Congenital infection possible in UK – where mother visited endemic area

Exclusion period
- Nil

Diagnosis
- Clinical + microscopy of fresh blood film

Management
- Drug treatment depends on type of infecting organism and resistance

Measles

- Organism – an RNA paramyxovirus
- Notifiable in the UK
- Vaccine available – routine immunization

Clinical summary
- Fever, conjunctivitis, gastroenteritis, coryza, cough, blotchy rash, Koplik spots
- Complications include otitis media, pneumonia, encephalitis, subacute sclerosing panencephalitis

Incubation period
- 8–13 days to fever
- 10–15 days to rash

Infectious period
- From first symptoms until 4 days after rash appears
- Low risk after 2 days of rash

Method of spread
- Droplet
- Highly infectious

Exclusion period
- Until 4 days after appearance of the rash

Diagnosis
- Clinical

Management
- Antipyretics + treatment of secondary infection
- Rapid immunization recommended for unimmunized contacts

Meningococcal disease

- Organism – *Neisseria meningitidis* – nine serotypes, B and C most prevalent in UK
- Notifiable in the UK
- Vaccine developed for groups A and C, e.g. foreign travel, case contacts – poor response in infants

Clinical summary
- Abrupt onset, fever, petechial rash, purpuric rash, meningitis, shock, collapse
- Also causes pneumonia, bacteraemia, septic arthritis, infective endocarditis

Incubation period
- Commonly 3–4 days (extreme range 2–10 days)

Infectious period
- Some patients continue to be infectious for a long time from mouth and nose discharges
- There are also carriers

Contacts
- Close family contacts are all treated with rifampicin and penicillin
- Group A and C contacts – vaccinate

Method of spread
- Droplet
- Moderately infectious

Exclusion period
- Seek advice

Diagnosis
- Clinical + microbiological (blood culture and CSF microscopy and culture)

Management
- Admit to hospital as emergency
- Intravenous antibiotics
- Treatment of complications
- Follow up to detect neurological problems, especially in most severely ill children

Meningitis from other causes

- Notifiable in the UK
- *Haemophilus influenzae; Streptococcus pneumoniae* (= 'pneumococcus')
  — Incubation period: 1–7 days
  — Infectious period: until 24 hours of antibiotics received
  — Diagnosis: bacteriological
  — Management: *Haemophilus* – ampicillin
                    Pneumococcus – penicillin
- Viral meningitis
  — Occurs in epidemics in young children in whom symptoms are variable
  — Incubation period: variable
  — Infectious period: until clinically recovered – infectivity high, but incidence of illness low
  — Diagnosis: CSF examination
  — Management: general supportive measures

Molluscum Contagiosum

- Organism – a poxvirus

Clinical summary
- Small pearly papules with central umbilication

Incubation period
- 2 to 7 weeks

Infectious period
- As long as lesions exist

Method of spread
- Very close contact
- Very low infectivity

Exclusion period
- None

Diagnosis
- Clinical

Management
- No treatment unless very severe or for cosmetic reasons
- Local application of trichloroacetic acid or phenol

Mumps

- Organism – a paramyxovirus
- Notifiable in the UK
- Vaccine available – routine immunization

Clinical summary
- Painful swelling of parotid or submandibular glands, may be unilateral

- General malaise and fever
- Complications include pancreatitis, sensorineural deafness, meningitis, orchitis in adults

Incubation period
- Commonly 18 days (extreme range 14–21 days)

Infectious period
- 6 days before swelling to 9 days after

Method of spread
- Droplet
- Low infectivity

Exclusion period
- For 7 days after swelling has appeared

Diagnosis
- Clinical

Management
- Symptomatic

Pneumonia

- Organisms
  - Bacterial: *Mycoplasma*; *Streptococcus pneumoniae* (= pneumococcus)
  - Viral
  - In young infant: *Chlamydia*, *Staphylococcus*, *Haemophilus* possible

Clinical summary
- Fever, respiratory distress, drowsiness or irritability
- Signs may be subtle in young children

Incubation period
- Variable

Infectious period
- Until bacteria eliminated or clinical recovery
- Spread of bacteria common, but illness in contacts rare

Method of spread
- Droplet

Exclusion
- For clinical reasons only

Management
- Hospitalization
- General measures
- Antibiotics: flucloxacillin + amoxycillin or erythromycin

Polio

- Organism – Enterovirus – three main types
- Notifiable in the UK (acute poliomyelitis)
- Vaccine available – routine immunization

Clinical summary
- Headache and sore throat leading in some cases to paralytic poliomyelitis

Incubation period
- Usually 7–14 days (extreme range 3–35 days)

Infectious period
- 3–6 weeks, via faeces

Method of spread
- Faeces → hand → mouth
- Highly infectious

Exclusion period
- Seek advice

Diagnosis
- Clinical + recovery of virus from throat swab and faeces; serology

Management
- General supportive measures
- Bed rest, respiratory support, physiotherapy

Respiratory syncytial virus

- Organism – an RNA paramyxovirus

Clinical summary
- Bronchiolitis, croup, URTI

Incubation period
- 5–8 days

Infectious period
- Days from onset of symptoms

Method of spread
- Droplet

Exclusion period
- Until asymptomatic

Diagnosis
- Clinical + virology

Management
- General supportive measures

Ringworm

- Organism – *Microsporum, Trichophyton, Epidermophyton* species

Clinical summary
- Ring-like lesions on body
- On scalp, accompanied by hair loss
- On feet there is scaling and maceration between the toes (athlete's foot)
- Nails dull, brittle, thickened, distorted, separated from nail bed

Incubation period
- Scalp – 10–14 days
- Body – 4–10 days
- Feet – unknown

Infectious period
- As long as lesions are present

Method of spread
- Direct contact
- Low infectivity

Exclusion period
- Scalp – until lesions are healing
- Body – none
- Feet – none

Diagnosis
- Clinical + mycology of skin scrapings/nail clippings
- Some species glow green in Wood's (UV) light

Management
- Generally topical, e.g. econazole, miconazole, clotrimazole
- Treatment should continue for 10 days after apparent cure to prevent recurrence
- Oral treatment (griseofulvin) needed for scalp/nail lesions, often for long periods

Roseola infantum (exanthem subitum, 'sixth disease')

- Organism – probably Human Herpes Virus 6

Clinical summary
- High fever with a discrete macular rash appearing on the trunk as the temperature drops and the child improves

Incubation period
- 10 days

Infectious period
- Unknown

Method of spread
- Close contact
- Moderately infectious

Exclusion period
- Nil

Diagnosis
- Clinical

Management
- Reduce temperature in view of risk of febrile convulsions

Rubella

- Organism – Rubella virus
- Notifiable in the UK
- Vaccine available – routine immunization

Clinical summary
- Fine, discrete maculopapular rash
- Fever, occipital lymphadenopathy
- Congenital rubella – serious damage to the fetus if infection occurs in first trimester of pregnancy (ophthalmological, cardiac, auditory, neurological)

Incubation period
- Usually 16–18 days (extreme range 14–23 days)

Infectious period
- From 7 days before rash until 4 days after

Method of spread
- Droplet or direct contact
- High infectivity

Exclusion period
- Until 4 days after appearance of rash
- Most important to isolate from non-immune pregnant women in first trimester

Diagnosis
- Clinical, but later immune status cannot be assumed as clinical picture mimicked by many other infections

Management
- General measures

Scabies

- Organism – *Sarcoptes scabiei* mite

Clinical summary
- Red papular rash in interdigital spaces, flexor surfaces of wrists, elbows, axillae and back
- Very itchy
- Burrows seen

Incubation period
- Days to weeks

Infectious period
- Until mites and eggs are destroyed

Method of spread
- Very close contact
- Low infectivity

Exclusion period
- Until after treatment has started

Diagnosis
- Clinical

Management
- Malathion (Prioderm, Derbac-M), Permethrin (Lyclear)
- Lindane (Quellada), avoid in young children, pregnant or breast-feeding mothers, history of epilepsy
- Aqueous preparations preferable
- Apply to whole body from neck down with brush, including webs of fingers and toes, and nails. Infants under 2 include scalp, neck, face, and ears
- Treat all family members at same time
- Itching can be controlled with calamine, crotamiton or antihistamines
- Only one application necessary if applied properly

Shigella (bacillary dysentery)

- Organism – *Shigella* bacteria – four groups
- Notifiable in the UK

Clinical summary
- Profuse diarrhoea (bloody), abdominal pain, fever, vomiting

Incubation period
- Commonly 1–3 days (extreme range 1–7 days)

Infectious period
- Usually only while symptomatic
- There are carriers

Method of spread
- Faeces → hand → mouth
- High infectivity
- Important in day nurseries
- Stress general hygiene
- Avoid closure if possible

Exclusion period
- Until 3 negative stool specimens are obtained (collected from separate visits to the toilet)

Diagnosis
- Stool culture

Management
- General measures to prevent dehydration
- Antibiotics and antidiarrhoeal agents are generally unnecessary and the former can prolong the carrier state

Streptococcal tonsillitis

- Organism – *Streptococcus pyogenes* (group A haemolytic) – many strains
- Scarlet fever notifiable in the UK

Clinical summary
- Follicular tonsillitis, fever, malaise, cervical lymphadenopathy
- May be associated scarlet fever
  - Punctate erythema desquamation
  - Strawberry tongue
  - Complications include rheumatic fever, chorea, glomerulonephritis

Incubation period
- 2–5 days

Infectious period
- Until 24 hours of treatment is complete

Method of spread
- Droplet

Exclusion period
- Until clinical recovery

Diagnosis
- Clinical + bacteriological

Management
- Penicillin for 10 days; erythromycin if penicillin sensitive

Other causes of tonsillitis/pharyngitis
- Other *Streptococcus* types, *Neisseria* species, *Haemophilus influenzae*
- Viruses – adenoviruses, enteroviruses, influenza and parainfluenza viruses

Tetanus

- Organism – *Clostridium tetani*
- Notifiable in the UK
- Vaccine available – routine immunization; wounds, depending on risk and previous cover

Clinical summary
- Pain, local then generalized muscle spasms

Incubation period
- Commonly 4–10 days (extreme range 4–21 days)

Infectious period
- No person to person spread

Method of spread
- From spores in soil into open wound, especially penetrating injuries and dirty wounds; also burns

Exclusion period
- Nil

Diagnosis
- History, clinical, microbiological

Management
- Surgical exploration and wound debridement, general measures, sedation
- Tetanus immunoglobulin, penicillin V
- Hospital treatment as emergency

Threadworms
- Organism – nematode worm *Enterobius vermicularis*

Clinical summary
- Pruritus ani, threads seen in stool or perianally – white worms 2–12 mm long
- May be asymptomatic

Incubation period
- Ingestion → egg laying 6 weeks

Infectious period
- As long as viable eggs present on body or in dust

Method of spread
- Female worm lays eggs on perianal skin → itching → scratching → eggs on fingers and under nails → mouth and spread to others
- Inhalation of dust containing eggs
- Eggs laid at night, then female usually dies
- Eggs can survive 2–3 weeks at room temperature
- 6 week life cycle, spontaneous resolution unless reinfected

Exclusion period
- Nil

Diagnosis
- Clinical, or ova seen on microscopy after collection on adhesive tape – may need several specimens, only 50% picked up on first specimen

Management
- Piperazine, two doses 1 week later
- Mebendazole, single dose, only children over 2
- Treat whole family at same time

- Reinfection common
- Hygiene important to prevent spread, especially scrubbing finger nails
- Damp dusting, frequent vacuuming

Tuberculosis

- Organism – *Mycobacterium* species
- Notifiable in the UK
- Vaccine available – routine Heaf testing and immunization of school children aged 10–13; other high-risk groups, e.g. immigrants from countries with high prevalence of TB and their children, contacts

Clinical summary
- Presentation highly variable
- Result of screening or contact tracing
- Sensitivity reaction
- Vague ill health
- Pulmonary symptoms
- Miliary disease: lethargy, fever, weight loss
- Meningitis
- Synovitis or osteitis
- Tonsillar infection
- Abdominal mass (very rare in UK)

Incubation period
- 4–12 weeks

Infectious period
- Variable, seek advice

Method of spread
- Close contact, droplet
- Low infectivity

Exclusion period
- Seek advice
- Usually non-infectious after 3 weeks of therapy

Diagnosis
- Clinical, tuberculin testing, radiology, microscopy and culture

Management
- Antituberculous chemotherapy

Typhoid

- Organism – *Salmonella typhi*
- Notifiable in the UK
- Vaccine available, e.g. foreign travel

Clinical summary
- Extreme malaise, fever, rose spots

- Usually mild in infants

Incubation period
- 1–3 weeks

Infectious period
- Until stools clear

Method of spread
- Faecal → hand → oral
- Food and water
- Moderately infectious

Exclusion period
- Seek advice

Diagnosis
- Isolation of organism from stool or blood culture, serology

Management
- Ampicillin or chloramphenicol
- General measures

Warts and verrucae

- Organism – Human Papilloma virus – several serotypes

Clinical summary
- Refer to text – page 146

Incubation period
- 4 months (extreme range 1–12 months)

Infectious period
- Unknown
- Possibly as long as lesion lasts

Method of spread
- Very close contact
- Infectivity very low

Exclusion period
- None

Diagnosis
- Clinical

Management
- See text – page 146
- For genital and peri-anal warts, consider sexual abuse

Whooping cough

- Organism – *Bordetella pertussis*
- Notifiable in the UK

- Vaccine available – routine immunization

Clinical summary
- Catarrhal prodromal illness leading to long lasting paroxysmal cough
- Typical whoop may be absent in children under one and those over 10

Incubation period
- Commonly 7–10 days (extreme range 7–21 days)

Infectious period
- Up to 3 weeks after paroxysmal coughing starts or until 7 days after antibiotic is commenced

Method of spread
- Droplet
- High infectivity

Exclusion period
- Until 5 days from starting antibiotic treatment

Diagnosis
- Clinical, lymphocytosis, per-nasal swab

Management
- Erythromycin, general nursing care
- Check immunization of contacts
- Give erythromycin for contacts under 6 months

NUTRITION

Infant feeding
- National (DH) and International (WHO, FAO) bodies have made recommendations on the nutritional requirements of infants and children. The figures shown on infant food containers have to conform to these recommendations. They all err on the high side and do not always acknowledge the wide individual variation
- Individuals vary widely in both total intake and in the frequency and regularity of feeds
- Adequacy of intake is best judged by evidence of normal growth and development

Analysis of feeding problems
- Feeding problems can be expressed as:
    — Anxiety that the infant is not getting enough
    — Concern that the milk does not suit (food sensitivity)
    — Regurgitation and vomiting
    — Frequent loose, foul smelling stools
    — Failure to thrive

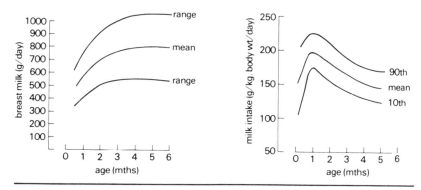

Fig. 4.13 Daily milk intake.

Table 4.6 Commonly used milk formulae

Highly modified	Premium	Cow and Gate
	SMA Gold	SMA nutrition
	First	Farley
	Aptamil	Milupa
	Formula 1	Boots
	First menu, first stage	Sainsbury
Modified	Plus	Cow and Gate
	SMA White	SMA nutrition
	Second	Farley
	Milumil	Milupa
	Formula 2	Boots
	First menu, second stage	Sainsbury
Vegetable-based	Infrasoy	Cow and Gate
	SMA Wysoy	SMA nutrition
	Prosbee powder	Mead Johnson
	OsterSoy	Farley
	(milk-free and lactose-free)	

- In an analysis of all of these it is important to make a general enquiry about the *food*, the *delivery system* and the *recipient*

The food
- What is the child receiving?
- Is it sufficient in amount?
- Are vitamin supplements needed?
- Parents may elect to feed their infant by the breast or by the bottle; they may choose to wean at 1 or 6 months – there are many routes to success
- The great majority of mothers should be encouraged to breast feed and to wean in the fourth month
- On peak production, a UK mother on 'average' produces about 800 ml a day, probably more than enough for the 'average' infant up to 4 months of age

Types of milk
Milk is a complete diet in one:
- There are four main alternatives for young babies:
  — Human milk
  — Highly modified cow's milk formula (casein/whey ratio 40:60)
  — Modified milk formula (casein/whey ratio 80:20 as in cow's milk)
  — Vegetable based formula (soy protein)
  — All others except special infant formula are unsuitable
- From 6 months, parents can use:
  — Breast milk or infant formula, listed above
  — Family dishes containing whole pasteurised cow's milk
  — Follow on milk
- From 1 year:
  — Whole pasteurized cow's milk
- The following are unsuitable for young children:
  — Skimmed and semi-skimmed milk
  — Goat's milk
- There are no important differences between milks in any one category, and changes in formula should be discouraged
- There are special infant formulae for infants with phenylketonuria, galactosaemia and severe malabsorption problems. They should not be used without expert dietetic advice
- There are also special feeds for preterm infants, but no infant should be discharged from hospital on such high density milk

Amount
- Requirements vary widely from 100–200 ml/kg/day (2.5 oz/lb/day)
- Check growth centile chart

Supplements
- All the artificial formulae to varying degrees are fortified with iron and vitamins, particularly vitamin D
  — The vitamin, iron and calcium contents are higher than those in breast milk
  — However, breast fed babies do not all require supplementation, but this is important where there are reasons for concern about maternal nutrition
  — Vitamin drops containing vitamins A, C, and D are available from clinics and are recommended up to the age of 5 in families where nutrition is likely to be poor

The delivery system
Problems with breasts and bottles
- The breasts may become engorged and painful
  — Requires analgesics and breast emptying
- The nipples may be sore and bleed
  — Requires rest and local creams
- Bottles may be difficult to clean
  — Requires advice and the correct facilities

- Teats may have holes that are too big so that the flow is too fast and the baby chokes, or too small so that the flow is too slow and the baby swallows air with the milk
  — Requires adjustment
- Infant feeds may, and often are, made too strong
  — Parents and nurses may be generous with the powder
  — If suspected, watch mother make a feed and counsel
- Too dilute feeds given over a period of time will provide an inadequate intake

The recipient
- Babies' appetites vary. Some are greedy and gobble; others are indifferent and nibble. Mothers usually know this, but may not appreciate how their infant differs from others
- Feeding difficulty may be the first indication of a variety of major problems from palatal cleft to heart disease and learning disability, so always check the baby over, and, if in doubt, watch the infant feed

Individual feeding problems

Mother's fear that she does not have enough milk or feels unable to satisfy her baby
- Ask about her physical well-being and diet
- Ask if she is tired, sleeps well or is inexplicably sad or moody
- Enquire about the feeding pattern
- And, if necessary, watch the baby feed
- Demonstrate weight gain on child's growth chart

It is rare for the breast or the baby to be the reason.

Management
- Support mother

Concern that the food does not suit
- Food intolerance means that the infant is unable to digest the food
- Food sensitivity means that the food upsets the infant either in the bowel or systemically
- Food allergy means that the infant has an allergic hypersensitivity to a food
  — All three have been confused and are not as common as some 'authorities' or artificial milk manufacturers would suggest
  — On the other hand, they do exist and for the few affected infants and their families they can be very upsetting
  — There is no alternative to taking a meticulous history of dietary intake and the timing, expression and course of the symptoms

Transient lactose intolerance
- Occurs after some episodes of gastroenteritis due to damage to the superficial layer of the bowel lining which contains the lactose disaccharidase

- Lactose found in the stool
- Is not usually severe enough to discontinue breast milk (100% carbohydrate in form of lactose)
- The lactose content of artificial cow's milk feeds varies between manufacturers
- Soy formulae are lactose-free

Infants who develop colic or rashes

- These are not in themselves grounds for experimenting with different feeds, but for making the right diagnosis

Infants with eczema or a strong family history of allergic disorders

- Breast feeding is generally recommended but is not protective
- Some question that infantile eczema is an allergic disorder
- Human breast milk can contain complex proteins from the mother's diet in minute amounts (including cow's milk protein)
- What the mother eats (prunes, curry) can upset the infant, so maternal diet will require consideration

Cow's milk hypersensitivity

- An infant develops a confluent perioral rash and swelling every time milk enters the mouth
- Others retch and vomit after a feed; the vomit may contain blood
- Occurs within hours of the feed, have colic and pass a loose, blood-streaked stool
- Others react with any combination of the three
- Soy feeds do not contain cow's milk protein and are the first alternatives to consider
- Infants can also become sensitive to soy protein
- Goat's milk is not recommended for infants

Regurgitating or vomiting feeds

- Note the feeding schedule and the time taken to feed
- Determine the timing of the reflux in relation to feed
- Is the baby eager to feed again?
- Estimate the volume lost
- Does his mother think the baby is uncomfortable?
- Is the vomit streaked with blood?
- Is the baby thriving?

Management
If, as is usually the case, the volume lost is small and the infant is thriving:

- Reassure parents that the infant is well
- Sympathize about the smell and the extra washing
- Counsel on feeding technique, particularly a quiet, firm, unhurried approach, giving baby the time to settle to and after the feed

If the vomit is considerable, but the baby is gaining weight:

- Consider thickening feeds

- Modified milk (casein/whey 80:20) will form thicker curds than highly modified formula or soy feed
- Thickening agents, which thicken the feed in the stomach, like cornflower thickens a sauce, may help, e.g. Carobel and arrowroot
- Avoid lying flat
- Older children can be positioned upright after feeds
- In the younger child, there is a growing body of opinion that the 30° prone position is preferable to the right lateral

If the vomit is very considerable, the baby is distressed or not gaining weight, then consider:
- Infection (urinary tract)
- Pyloric stenosis
- Hiatus hernia
- Severe child–parent dysharmony

Frequent foul-smelling stools
The threshold of parents' anxiety varies
- Stools may be passed with each feed or every other day
- They may vary from liquid green to chalky yellow
- They rarely smell pleasant; they all smell worse when mixed with urine and after keeping (especially at 37°C between the buttocks!)
- Toddlers' stools often contain undigested food – peas, carrot cubes etc.

Reassure unless:
- There has been sudden and recent change
    — Exclude infection and check what has been swallowed
- The baby is off colour, dehydrated or has a fever
    — Seek underlying causes
- The infant is failing to thrive

Toddler diarrhoea is a recognised entity:
- It may result from over-feeding, an excessive gastro-colic reflex or be a phase in the development of large-bowel function
- Usually requires reassurance only, but can be helped with loperamide in severe cases

'Failure to thrive'
This label embraces a variety of entities:
- A slow growing but otherwise healthy infant
- An underfed healthy infant
- An underloved but reasonably fed infant
- A chronically sick infant
- An ill-formed or brain damaged infant
- An infant with malabsorption

The distinction can usually be made on the basis of:
- Clinical history of infant
- Social history
- Enquiry of infant–parent relationship

- Physical examination
- Previous weight charts

Management seeks to answer the following questions:
- Is the child being offered enough of an appropriate food?
- Is the child able to take sufficient food?
- Is the child losing excessive amounts of food energy in urine or stools?
- Is the child using excessive amounts of food energy?

Action depends on the cause or causes; often more than one factor is involved

Follow-on milks and weaning

- There are many ways to wean infants, and in the UK it is difficult to get it wrong
- Food technology is now such that the range of foods that can be manufactured is virtually limitless
- 'Follow-on' milks are artificial milks, specially formulated for the toddler (such as milk shakes for older children)
- They must not be used as the only feed for young infants
- In essence, they have added protein, vitamins and iron
- They are not necessary; some may consider that they are not desirable either

Pre-school and school children – the fat and the thin

- Assessment of nutritional status in a growing child is not easy
- You may find it helpful to record:
  — Whether you think the child looks thin or fat
  — Whether there is a lot or little subcutaneous fat
  — Whether there is a lot or little muscle bulk
  — The condition of the skin, hair and signs of iron or calcium deficiency
  — The presence and extent of dental caries
  — Record and plot the child's weight and height
- Analysis of height/weight ratios by whatever formula, are helpful, but do not correlate well with nutritional intake or well-being and must be viewed within the cultural and genetic background
- More note might perhaps be taken of the child's feeling; is he or she:
  — Hungry?
  — Energetic or listless?
  — Enthusiastic or apathetic?

Management
If there is concern:
- Enquire about the child's eating habits
- Analyse the child's dietary intake
- Obtain reports on child's liveliness
- Assess growth increment
- If necessary, exclude iron-deficiency anaemia

- If the child is under-weight, under-sized or thin, counsel on appropriate changes in eating pattern and chosen foods
  — The adolescent with anorexia nervosa can be very devious
- If the child is over-weight and fat, likewise counsel on appropriate changes in eating patterns and chosen foods, but this time directed at reducing calorie intake
  — The obese child can also be very manipulative
- For both problems, concentration on food alone is unwise; the aim should be to encourage a healthier lifestyle, of which eating and food are only a part

Food refusal
- Refuse solids – spit/vomit it out. Prefers milk
- Usually in toddlers who were weaned late ± associated behaviour concerns
- May be associated with iron-deficiency anaemia
- Diagnosis of exclusion – *rarely*, significant gastro-esophageal reflux/neurological disorders which impair swallowing or abdominal pain secondary to food intolerance

Management
- Exclude serious disorders and treat if iron-deficient
- Reassure parent
- Behaviour programme for meal times

Obesity
Pre-school child
- History as above – include parental perceptions and influences from grandparents
- Obese pre-schoolers may improve spontaneously by adolescence with no intervention
- Important to establish 'healthy eating' programme if possible and enquire about sugar intake as dental hygiene is of paramount importance

School-aged child
- History as above
- Most are aware of their obesity
- Try to target children with a body mass index above the 90th centile (see chart in appendix)
- They have an increased tendency to remain obese into adulthood
- Obtain perception of both child and parents. They may *not* want intervention

Plan
- Dietary history (food diary, including drinks and 'snacks') and any routine exercise
- Be aware that both may be inaccurate as most people naturally remember their most healthy activities. Snacks are forgotten and

food portions which are larger than normal may be considered 'average'

- *Do not be pejorative* – any indication that they are 'at fault' for being obese can alienate them, regardless of how well meaning you may otherwise appear
- Explain need for maintenance of static weight – usually an easier objective than weight loss. Use growth charts and BP measurements to support argument but:
- Try *not* to focus purely upon above. Explain possibility of bullying and explore self-esteem. This may be a very important factor in young people who fail to lose or control weight
- Engage parents in importance of improving self-esteem in their children if it is an issue
- Intervention should be intensive:
    - Initial consultation with school nurse ± doctor then monthly sessions for another three sessions
    - Do *not* discuss weight at all sessions, can be demoralising or intimidating. Start with positive points, i.e. holiday
    - Make plan clear at start of programme
    - Healthy eating and *regular* exercise which suits the child – not what you feel should be done
    - Ensure 'healthy food' can still be 'fun' – get parents to try to be imaginative if possible (recipes from magazines)
    - Not to spend excessive money on 'special diet'
    - *Family* should have the same meals or child will again be alienated
    - If the child agrees, try to get them to bring a single close friend to the sessions for continuing moral support – friend need not be obese
    - Review progress after the six sessions. If *not* progressing – STOP and suggest child/teenager contact you if they want to try again. Aim to empower them/families as opposed to 'driving them to stay healthy'
    - Select candidates for programme carefully. Your time is precious and limited!

CHILD PROTECTION

Definition of child abuse: 'any intended or unintended act or omission which adversely affects the child's health, physical growth or psychosocial development, whether or not regarded by the child or adult as abusive'

Four main types:

- Physical
- Sexual

- Emotional
- Neglect

These categories are not mutually exclusive, and it is estimated that one-third of children who have been sexually abused have also been subjected to physical abuse in addition.

Each District has a child protection register (CPR) which is held by social services and aids monitoring of child abuse for both individual cases and to look at trends within a population.

Purposes of the CPR:

- To provide a record of all children in the district with unresolved child protection issues and for whom there is in place an interagency child protection plan
- To maintain a record of and answer enquiries made about children where there are suspicions of abuse
- To facilitate communication and coordination between agencies and individual workers
- To provide management information for the Area Child Protection Committee (ACPC)

Prevalence in children, 0–15 years, of all forms of abuse (statistics from CPRs in England 1993):

- 4.4/1000 boys
- 4.6/1000 girls

< 1 year	7%
1–4 years	31%
5–9 years	32%
10–15 years	27%
16–17 years	4%

(Grave concern 34% (no longer included as a category); physical injury 28%; neglect 19%; sexual abuse 17%; emotional abuse 7%)

1 in 10 adult women admit to having been sexually abused at some stage in their childhood or adolescence and may present with multiple difficult symptomatology to different doctors.

The doctor's role
- Early identification and appropriate referral by prompt detection of abnormal or suspicious history and physical examination findings
- Prevention by recognition of risk factors for the different forms of abuse and modifying these where possible
- Liaison with social services, police, probation, health visitors, teachers, general practitioners and hospital staff
- Surveillance of copies of hospital letters, notes from Accident Departments

- Recognised as an area of paediatrics which doctors may find very difficult and upsetting personally. Access to senior advice is essential for support

- All doctors should familiarize themselves with the official child protection procedures in their locality
- Recognised risk factors
  — Parents themselves abused or in care as children
  — Families under stress (relationship difficulties, milestones, e.g. births, leaving home, deaths)
  — Maternal or paternal learning difficulties (often useful to ask about parental schooling)
  — Maternal illness, particularly mental illness (asking: 'have you ever had any problems with your 'nerves'?' is one way of ascertaining this)
  — Premature and low birthweight infants
  — Early separation from infant (e.g. early hospitalization)
  — Parental drug dependence
  — Criminality in the family (particularly violent crime) highly predictive
  — Poor socio-economic circumstances
  — Young parents
  — Parental smoking
- In all cases there are three main tasks involved for the doctor faced with a child protection case:
  — OBSERVE
  — RECORD CAREFULLY
  — REPORT APPROPRIATELY

Physical abuse

- The following circumstances are classically associated with inflicted injury
- They are not, however, diagnostic
  — No explanation or inadequate explanation of injuries
  — Delay in seeking medical help
  — Changing explanation for injury
  — Different explanations from different people
  — Recurrent injuries in child or sibling
  — Injuries that could not have occurred simultaneously

History
- Complete
- Careful
- Of injury
  — When
  — Where
  — How
  — Time from incident to caretaker seeking help or to others expressing concern
  — Witnesses

- Of child
  - Age
  - Previous injuries
  - Significant life events
  - Developmental history
  - General health
  - Is child on Local Child Protection Register?
  - Have there been other register enquiries about the child? (telephone yourself – number in local child protection procedures)
- Of family
  - Composition – family tree and genogram
  - Household
  - Other contacts with children
  - Family supports
  - Agencies involved – 'professionogram'
- Of environment
  - Type of accommodation/state of accommodation
  - School

Examination
- The child's injuries (precise description needed)
  - Length, width, position, colour, shape
  - Bruises, how well demarcated?
  - Burns – position, shape
    Use diagrams – it is better to use standard body maps where possible. These may be supplemented by photographs taken by the medical photography department or police photographers. Polaroid photographs may be useful as a supplement to the records, but do not make as accurate a copy of injuries as professional photographs.
- The rest of the child
  - General appearance, cleanliness, state of clothes
  - Length/height and weight plotted on percentile chart with previous measurements
  - General affect – frozen watchfulness, apathy
- In particular
  - Examine the whole child
  - Scalp and hair – any missing?
  - Ears – bruised, swollen, torn tympanic membranes, look behind pinna for hidden marks
  - Eyes – retinal haemorrhages
  - Mouth – gum damage, torn frenulum
  - Neck – bruises
  - Genitalia, anus
- Parent–child interaction
  - Parents showing appropriate concern

— Relationship between parent and child
— Child's behaviour
- Date and sign your documentation as it may be legal evidence

Specific injuries

Bruises
- May 'track' along tissue planes
- Deep-seated bruises may take days to reach the surface
- Bruises must be differentiated from mongolian blue spots which may present anywhere on the body and are occasionally found in children of apparently fair skinned stock
- Colour progression
  — Red/violet – initially
  — To blue/purple/black after 1–3 days
  — To green/yellow/brown – usually at least 3 days old
  — Yellowing and fading – 7–14 days
  — Resolved in 2–4 weeks
- Age is hard to tell and is more difficult if the skin is naturally pigmented
- Doctor should state that bruise is consistent with being X days old rather than giving any categorical age as wide variation occurs
- Features suggesting bruising due to physical abuse
  — Multiple bruises at different sites
  — Bruises of different ages
  — Fingertip bruises (check for pattern of fingers)
  — Well demarcated linear bruises (due to sharp object hitting child)
  — Slap marks
  — Black eyes – particularly bilateral (be wary that blood from forehead injury may track down to soft tissues around the eyes)
  — Teeth marks (crescentic bruises are characteristic)
  — Bruises on legs of child who is not yet walking
  — Bruises to the face and neck after 3 years of age
  — Bruises to the lower back of a child under 3 years of age
  — Bruises to perianal, umbilical or vaginal areas

Burns and scalds
- Features suggestive of non-accidental origin
  — Contact burns in abnormal sites
  — Glove and stocking scalds to hands and feet (suggestive of forcible immersion in hot water)
  — Repeated burns incompatible with history
  — Burns to back of hand or wrist (punishment)
  — Any well demarcated burn without an explanation
  — 'Cigarette burns' – well demarcated round deep burns especially on hands, wrist or face. (Cigarette burns can be accidental but these are usually single, superficial, elliptical lesions due to brief contact)
  — Impetigo should be considered in the differential diagnosis

Neglect

- Parents fail to provide the child's basic needs
- Occasionally malevolent
- More often associated with low income, parents' incapacity due to mental illness/alcohol
- Poor parenting skills (parents themselves abused, neglected or institutionalized)
- Parental low intelligence
- Food
  — Insufficient calories
  — Classical growth disturbance; weight more affected than height, head circumference spared
  — Unbalanced, disorganized, irregular calories, e.g. prolonged milk feeds producing iron deficiency, diets of crisps and sweets
  — Must exclude organic disease, e.g. coeliac, malrotation
  — Calorie neglect and organic disease may co-exist
- Warmth
  — Of housing – related to finances and type of house
  — Of clothing – dressed inappropriately for season
- Cleanliness
  — Standards of 'normal' hygiene vary
  — Prolonged contact with an unchanged nappy will cause an erosive ammoniacal dermatitis
  — Recurrent gastroenteritis due to poor bottle sterilization and hand washing
  — Impetigo, excoriation of upper lip due to un-cleaned constantly running nose
- Health
  — Incomplete immunization for no good reason
  — Failure to recognise illness
  — Failure to complete necessary treatment
- Safety
  — Failure to child-proof the home e.g.
    Fireguards
    Poisons out of reach
    Stair and garden gates
    Appropriate car seating
- Emotions
  — Lack of normal interaction with adults, e.g. locked up or left alone in cot and rarely picked up or spoken to
  — Multiple caretakers with little commitment to the child
  — Maternal mental illness
- Education
  — Play space
  — Toys (though cultural norms vary)
  — Lack of visual stimulation

— Absence from school (older children)
— Inappropriate television viewing (video nasties)

Examination
- Affect
  — Inappropriate for age
  — Lack of eye contact in infancy
  — 'Radar' gaze when older
  — Lack of stranger fear in a toddler – will go to anyone to be picked up
  — Abnormal socialization in pre-school child – inability to interact with peers
- Development
  — Delayed, particularly speech and language
  — Poverty of play
- Physical
  — Growth abnormalities – wasting of buttocks
  — Anaemia
  — Dental caries
  — Chronic suppurative otitis media
  — Impetigo
  — Contact dermatitis
  — Smell of stale urine
  — Cold thin limbs
  — Pink puffy 'deprivation hands and feet'
  — Thin sparse hair
  — Loss of hair from occiput
- Growth charts
  — Regular monitoring of growth is vital in suspected neglect
  — Try to use same scales – again very important in court case
  — Calibrate scales
  — Naked weights
  — Plot measurements – charts need to have each point signed to be admissible in court
  — Do not forget length measurement (supine until 2 years of age, standing when older than 2 years)

Sexual abuse
- 1 in 10 girls and 1 in 15 boys under the age of 16 will be sexually assaulted
- Peak age is 8 but occurs at all ages
- 80% are abused by someone known to them
- Sexual abuse has a prolonged time course: secrecy, guilt, loss of trust and lack of self esteem are its hallmarks

Highly suspicious signs
- Pregnancy under 16 (particularly where father is not disclosed)
- Venereal disease, including anal/vaginal warts

- Childhood disclosure to friend/teacher/parent
- Genital trauma
- Abusing other children

General signs (not diagnostic but associated)
- Unexplained emotional disturbance
- Self-destructive behaviour
- Running away from home
- Sexual precocity
- Vague vaginal complaints
- Vaginal discharge
- Recurrent urinary/abdominal symptoms

History
- Approach depends upon age and manner of disclosure
- Should be taken fully by one person whom the child trusts
- Avoid repetitive history taking thereafter
- Note child's words verbatim
- Do not use leading questions
- Drawings or anatomically correct dolls will help – only to be used by expert in disclosure work
- Ascertain the child's particular words for bodily parts and functions
- Reassure the child 'this is not your fault'
- Beware separated parents using accusation of sexual abuse to attack the other partner

Examination
- Features suggestive of abuse may be found in a very young or otherwise well child
- If strongly suspected, then full examination should be carried out by an expert police surgeon or paediatrician in a specially equipped facility
  - It should not be carried out half-heartedly in the community
  - Body maps and detailed perineal views are useful for recording findings
- The following should be looked for:
  - Vagina
    Warts
    Discharge
    Torn hymen
    Dilated hymenal opening (>5 mm in a prepubertal girl)
  - Anus (commonest penetration in girls under 5 years)
    External haematoma or warts
    Peri-anal thickening
    Tears, especially multiple
    Short anal canal and proximity of anorectal junction to the external orifice
- Long-term effects
  - After disclosure the child may have to give evidence in court (the use of videotape has begun to eliminate this need)

— Family support will be necessary
— Long-term behavioural problems may result
  Self destructive behaviour
  'Post traumatic syndrome'
  Soiling and enuresis

Child protection legal framework

- Children Act 1989 in England and Wales – became operational in 1991. Similar laws apply in Scotland and Northern Ireland
- The Act replaced many different pieces of complex legislation affecting child care
- Overriding principle of the Act is to ensure the welfare of the child at all times and Courts have a checklist to ensure that this is upheld
- Parental responsibility replaces parental duties and rights. Parents who are married both have parental responsibility. An unmarried father can acquire it by mother's consent or where granted by the Court
- Parental responsibility carries the right to determine:
  — Where the child lives
  — How he/she is educated
  — The duty to care for the child
- Responsibility may pass to the local authority or a guardian in certain circumstances – important when considering consent for procedures such as immunization or surgical operations
- The community paediatrician needs to be familiar with the different 'Sections' of the Act particularly Sections 17 and 47

Section 17 describes the duty of the local authority to provide services for children 'in need'. A child is *in need* if:
- He is unlikely to achieve or maintain a reasonable standard of health or development without the provision of services (day care, accommodation, family aides, occupational therapy)
- His health or development is likely to be significantly impaired, or further impaired without the provision of services, or
- He is disabled (see section on Disability Register)
  Health is defined to mean physical or mental health, and development to mean physical, intellectual, emotional, social or behavioural development

These children may be chronic non-attenders at hospital and other appointments, within homeless or very mobile families. Young carers of disabled adults are a particularly vulnerable group at risk.

Many children are identified from the routine child health surveillance programme.

Section 47 states that the local authority has a duty to investigate situations where there is reasonable cause to suspect that a child *is suffering, or likely to suffer, significant harm* and take action to ensure the safety or promotion of a child's welfare.

- A doctor or other suspecting child abuse would use this section of the law to initiate an investigation by social services
- The Courts may issue a number of Orders under the Children Act following investigation including:
  — **Care Order** – places the child in the care of the local authority and confers parental responsibility (lasts until the child is 18 years unless discharged earlier)
  — **Supervision Order** – similar to above, but a medical or psychiatric examination may be requested during the period (lasts up to 1 year)
- The doctor may be asked to provide evidence from a review of the child's health and development as to whether harm has occurred or is likely to occur
  — **Emergency Protection Order** (EPO) – can be applied for by anyone where the child is in immediate risk of harm and needs to be removed from a dangerous situation or prevented from being removed from a safe situation, e.g. in hospital or foster care (lasts for 8 days and can be extended by a further 7 days)
  — **Child Assessment Order** (CAO) – granted in non-urgent cases where the investigation to establish the facts requires assessment which is refused by the parents (lasts 7 days). A plan of assessment has to be presented to the Courts and has to be completed within the time scale

There are four special orders which can be attached to the above designed to solve specific problems and are for a specified period
Section 8 Orders:
- **A residence order** – sets out arrangements defining with whom a child is to live and confirms parental responsibility
- **A contact order** – requires the person with whom the child lives to allow contact with the person named in the order
- **A specific issue order** – gives directions whereby a particular question needs to be answered, e.g. directing the parent to allow the child medical investigation or treatment
- **A prohibited steps order** – prevents a step that would normally be covered by parental responsibility from being taken

Child abuse investigation procedure (UK)

- All UK Health Districts have written guidelines for community doctors which will be similar to those given below
- It is essential that you familiarize yourself with them

An example of hospital and community medical staff procedures

Hospital and community medical staff working within the health authority for the protection of children must be committed to full cooperation in working together with other Agencies. Every attempt should be made to:

- Accommodate the child's wishes in relation to the gender of the examining doctor wherever the service allows
- Meet the needs of the child and the family in providing a worker of the same race/culture and in terms of communication, a person who speaks the first language of the family
- Have sensitivity to any special needs of the child, e.g. learning or physical difficulties

Physical abuse

Where there is any suspicion that a child has suffered physical abuse, the child should be referred immediately for the specialist opinion of a paediatrician. Where the paediatrician's conclusion is that there has been physical abuse or the child is at risk of abuse:

- The duty officer for the social service department in the area where the child resides, or hospital social worker, should be informed immediately (out of office hours ring emergency duty team)
- The parents must be kept informed of the proceedings being undertaken in the interests of the child
- In the hospital units, in the unlikely event of the child being removed against advice while waiting to be seen, and before a paediatrician has seen the child, the matter should be discussed by telephone with the paediatrician who will decide whether it should be referred immediately to the duty social worker in the area where the child resides, or hospital social worker. (Out of office hours ring emergency duty team.) The senior nurse on call should be informed
- The paediatrician should be available to present medical evidence in court after 72 hours should an emergency protection order be sought or challenged

Where sexual abuse is suspected

Either as a result of the child physical abuse examination or as a result of an examination for some other purpose or for other reasons such as a child's behaviour or symptoms: the social services department should be contacted as above. The circumstances, such as the child being in A/E, or the police holding a suspect may make the medical examination urgent and precede joint interviews.

If there is uncertainty as to whether particular behaviour or appearance relates to sexual abuse refer to a paediatrician.

Where there is a clear allegation or disclosure of child sexual abuse:
- Accurate recordings should be made of the account of the allegation or disclosure and by whom and any comment offered by the child, or the account of any other concerns
- The child's demeanour should be noted, but the child should not be exposed to direct questioning regarding the allegation
- The social services department should be contacted. Sexual abuse procedures differ from physical abuse procedures and consist of:
  — A joint initial assessment interview by police and social services in order to prevent the child from being exposed to repeated interviews

— A medical examination where appropriate
— The subsequent calling of a child protection case conference

Neglect and emotional abuse

Where there is concern about adequacy or appropriateness of parenting:

- The doctor should obtain further relevant information from nursing colleagues; from within the department; health visitor, school nurse, general practitioner in the community; hospital paediatrician, Accident and Emergency department, and should re-assess the initial concern in the light of any information received
- If the concern remains apparent, the information should be passed to the duty social worker in the area where the child resides, or hospital social worker. The emergency duty team may need to be informed if the situation becomes urgent
- Accurate notes should be made of all concerns in the child's medical records, including interpretation of weight, growth and developmental charts; good quality photographs should be obtained, if appropriate

Case conference

Wherever possible doctors involved in seeing the child should attend the child protection case conference. A written report should be prepared and sent to social services regarding any incident and relevant aspects of his/her knowledge of the child and family.

A case conference should normally be held within 8 working days of referral and certainly within 15 days unless there are special circumstances recorded by the child protection coordinator or children's service manager.

Case reviews

Whenever a case involves an incident leading to the death of a child where child abuse is confirmed or suspected, or a child protection issue likely to be of major public concern arises, there will be an individual review by each agency and a composite review by the area child protection committee. Medical staff involved in such cases must cooperate with a health authority review and with any inter-agency review required by the area child protection committee.

History and circumstances

- History of family
- Place in family tree
- Composition of household
- Other professionals involved with the children
- Family medical conditions
- Family accommodations and supports
- School circumstances
- History of child (best from someone who knows the child well)
- Age, medical and developmental history

- Significant life events
- Previous injuries/hospital admissions
- General health, recent symptoms or illness, medicines
- Is child on child protection register?
- Have there been other register enquiries about the child?
- Circumstances
- Adequacy and completeness of explanation for injuries or assault
- Any delay in seeking medical help
- Changing explanations or different explanations from different people
- Recurring injuries in child or sibling
- Injuries that could not have occurred simultaneously

Standard examination will normally include:
Examination of the whole child with comments on:
- General appearance, cleanliness, state of clothes, length/height, head circumference and weight plotted on percentile charts with previous measurements, if known
- Interactions with parents and staff
- General emotional state and development
- In particular, scalp and hair where injuries may be hidden
- Behind ears, ear canals and drums
- Eyes for conjunctival haemorrhage and ophthalmoscopic search for retinal haemorrhage
- Mouth, particularly for gum or tooth damage, torn frenulum
- Face and neck for fine bruises
- Ribs for bruising, swelling, tenderness of fractures
- Arms and legs for grip marks, ligature marks; palms and soles
- Abdomen for bruises or internal damage
- Genitalia inspection of penis, scrotum, anus, vulva, urethra and hymen
- Document the child's injuries in precise detail: length, widths, positions, colour, shape, definition, character, age; use diagrams, plus photographs of injuries where possible
- Arrange for any X-rays or blood clotting tests that are necessary
- Contemporaneous legible hand-written notes with date and signature; summary and conclusions that agree with verbal reports
- Typed or hand-written report for social services within 72 working hours

Where sexual abuse is suspected
The medical examination is best done jointly by a paediatrician and police surgeon where staffing permits, so that any forensic evidence can be preserved and repeat examinations avoided. However, the essential feature is that the doctor performing the examination should have experience and training in the examination of sexually abused children. A complete examination will be done as described in the physical abuse section with the difference that the child will not usually be asked to repeat the story of abuse if this information has already been gathered in police and social work interviews.

In addition:
- The examination of the genitalia and anus will be undertaken in more detail
- Swabs may be taken to check for infection
- Forensic samples may be taken
- Instruments are only occasionally needed to inspect beyond the anus or hymen. This might occur in a post-pubertal child. A pre-pubertal child needing internal examination (e.g. after injury or rape) may necessitate special arrangements for a general anaesthetic.

Medico-legal reports/appearance in court

- It is best to have an experienced doctor go over any report you write for Court purposes
- It is advisable to have a practice session giving evidence to ensure that your notes are in order, readily available for scrutiny, and your manner checked

URINARY TRACT INFECTIONS

- Accurate diagnosis, prompt treatment, careful follow-up and investigation of urinary tract infection in childhood is essential
- In children under the age of 7 years, unrecognised and untreated bacteriuria and vesico-ureteric reflux result in permanent renal scarring and later risk of hypertension or impaired renal function

Symptoms and signs

History

Infants
- Misery, poor feeding, vomiting, failure to thrive, prolongation or recurrence of jaundice, pyrexia
- In boys history of a poor urinary stream highly suggestive of posterior urethral valves

Toddlers
- Unexplained high fever, abdominal pain, febrile convulsions

Pre-school and older child
- Dysuria, frequency, secondary enuresis, daytime wetting, fever possibly with rigors, loin pain, haematuria

At any age
- Fever, vomiting, haematuria, hypertension
- Constipation, threadworms, irritants and bubble baths predispose to bacteriuria
- Sexual abuse may be associated with symptoms of urinary tract infection

- Family history of urinary tract infection, or renal abnormalities, e.g. vesico-ureteric reflux, increases the likelihood of similar lesions being found

Examination
- Check for pyrexia, anaemia and hypertension
- Examine the abdomen for localized tenderness, renal masses, an enlarged bladder, constipation
- Look for neurological problems, suggested by abnormal gait, abnormal ankle reflexes, cutaneous abnormalities over the lower spine
- If there are local symptoms or recurrence of infections, the genitalia should be examined for local lesions and congenital abnormalities
- Dysmorphic features may indicate the possibility of a syndrome which includes renal abnormalities

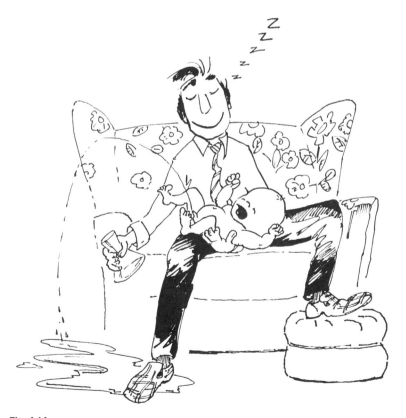

Fig. 4.14

Diagnosis

Urine samples
- Diagnosis of urinary infection and interpretation of results depends upon careful collection and transport of specimens
  - 20% of children with dysuria and frequency do not have bacterial urinary tract infections and can be spared unnecessary investigation if correct procedures are followed
- When collecting specimens, genitalia should be clean, but antiseptic scrubbing is unnecessary
- Once collected, specimens should be promptly transferred to sterile containers
- All specimens should get to the microbiology laboratory the same day if possible, and within 4 hours if microscopy is required
- If there is to be a delay of more than 6 hours, store specimen in refrigerator

Methods of collection
- Mid-stream urine (MSU)
  - Suitable for older continent children
- Clean-catch urine (CCU)
  - Method of choice in younger children
  - Requires an alert, patient person to collect it
  - Tapping over the bladder or the application of a cold object may provoke micturition
- Bag urine
  - Used in younger children, where clean-catch ineffective
  - Requires a carefully applied bag with infant held sitting and ideally no nappy, so that as soon as urine is passed, it can flow into the lower chamber and the bag can be removed, minimizing perineal contamination
  - Urine must not be decanted back through the entry hole – there is either a tab to pull or a hole should be cut in a dependent corner
  - Negative result is reliable; positive result should ideally be confirmed by clean-catch or supra-pubic specimen
- Supra-pubic aspirate (SPA)
  - Only for use in experienced hands when previous results are equivocal

Criteria for diagnosis
- UTI confirmed if pure growth of $>10^5$ bacteria per millilitre
- Pyuria (>10 white blood cells per millilitre) is usually found in the presence of acute symptoms but is not diagnostic
- Absence of pus cells or the presence of a mixed growth of bacteria is evidence against, but does not exclude, infection – repeat, or consider SPA

Nitrite test
- Reliable sign of infection when positive

- Up to 48% false-negative rate alone, 0% when combined with leucocytes (dipstix)
- Urine must have been in the bladder for at least 1 hour, so that there is time for bacterial conversion of nitrate to nitrite

Likely pathogens
- *Escherichia coli (E. coli)*
- *Klebsiella*
- *Proteus*
- *Streptococcus faecalis*
- *Staphylococcus epidermidis*, which is a pathogen in sexually active women and is usually a contaminant in children

Investigation and management

Investigation/referral
- All children under the age of 7 years should be referred to a paediatrician or paediatric nephrologist
  — 40% will be found to have vesico-ureteric reflux
  — 25% will be found to have renal scars
- Children over 7 years
  — Plain abdominal X-ray and renal ultrasound – refer if abnormality
  — Refer if recurrent infections
- Imaging studies required in all children with confirmed urinary tract infection
  — Protocols will depend upon age of child and local practice
  — May involve abdominal X-ray, ultrasound, intravenous urogram, micturating cysto-urethrogram, DMSA scan

Management
- Treatment should be started immediately if UTI clinically suspected, after appropriate sample of urine has been collected, with 'best guess' antibiotic
- Antibiotics should given/changed according to sensitivity results, for a course of 5–7 days
- Check for eradication of infection by sending a follow-up urine sample after completion of antibiotics
- Management of recurrent infections, underlying abnormalities and complications by appropriate specialist teams
  — Surgery
  — Regular/patient initiated urine cultures
  — Prophylactic antibiotics
  — Monitoring renal scarring/renal function

General measures to reduce the risk of recurrent infection and genital soreness in girls:
- Encourage regular bladder emptying
- Encourage double micturition
- Treat constipation

- Avoid tight trousers
- Bath regularly, dry carefully afterwards
- Avoid highly scented soap; do not use bubble bath or wash hair in bath
- Wipe bottom clean from front to back
- Use soft absorbent toilet paper
- Ensure easy access to satisfactory toilets in school
- Treat thrush and threadworms
- Discourage masturbation

DIABETES – ADVICE TO TEACHERS

- Nearly all children with diabetes will attend normal schools
- The few exceptions are due to social or emotional problems rather than the diabetes itself
- The child should carry glucose with him in case of hypoglycaemia
- A teacher should be aware of how to use hypostop (glucose gel rubbed into buccal mucosa) or i.m. glucogen; it is advantageous for fellow pupils to also be aware of this and the symptoms below
- The teacher needs to know the early symptoms:
  - — Confusion, poor work
  - — Trembling, sweating, weakness
  - — Drowsiness, headache
  - — Numbness and tingling
  - — Blurring of vision
  - — Abnormal gait
  - — Abnormal behaviour
  - — Loss of consciousness and convulsions are late symptoms
- The child with symptoms of hypoglycaemia should not be left alone until fully recovered
- He/she may need a snack outside the normal school timetable, e.g. on daily basis or before games or PE
- A suitable school dinner can nearly always be provided, though a packed lunch from home is an alternative
- School lunches should be served promptly and if there is an unusual delay, a snack should be offered
- The child with diabetes can take part in school outings and holidays, but the effects of changes in routine should be anticipated and discussed; decisions are based on the age of the child, his degree of self-sufficiency in terms of injections etc. and the availability and willingness of teachers to supervise

ADVICE TO SCHOOLS ON CHILDREN WITH CONGENITAL HEART DISEASE

- Children with heart disease rarely require any restriction
- Teachers may be anxious and require reassurance and explanation

- In severe cases, children will restrict themselves within their exercise tolerance
- Only children with aortic stenosis require restrictions; this should be carefully worked out with the school to avoid excessive measures being taken

HAEMOPHILIA

- Haemophilia is an X-linked recessive disorder caused by deficiency of factor VIII
- There are about 5000 cases in all in the UK
- Mild or moderate haemophiliacs will only encounter bleeding problems associated with surgery and severe injuries
- Severely affected haemophiliacs may bleed spontaneously into joints or muscles
- Currently used preparations are treated and screened for HIV and hepatitis B to minimize the risk of infection
- All haemophiliacs are screened for HIV and hepatitis and should have been immunized against hepatitis B

Advice to schools
- General
    — In general a boy with haemophilia should be treated quite normally in school and can take part in all activities, including PE, games (except contact sports), swimming, music lessons, including use of wind instruments, and other practical activities
    — School outings should not be barred as the parents should have a list of other haemophilia centres in the UK, all of which would be able to deal with any problems that might arise
- Small superficial cuts and grazes
    — Wash with soap and water and apply an adhesive water-proof dressing
    — The staff member should wear disposable gloves as with any other child
- Advice on dealing with any minor blood loss as with any other child
    — Advice intended to take proper precautions to prevent HIV
    — If blood is spilled, household bleach 1:10 should be applied to the spillage (not to the child!) and left for 30 minutes; disposable gloves should be worn, and disposable towels that can be flushed down the lavatory used to mop up
- Spontaneous internal bleeds into joints or muscles
    — With no external bleeding and therefore no risk of infection but should be treated seriously
    — Bleeding may be suspected if:
        Child complains that limb or joint 'feels funny'
        Reluctant to use limb or joint
        Complains of stiffness in limb or joint

There is swelling

Pain in limb or joint

The school should contact the parents to arrange *prompt* transfer to the haemophilia centre or for home treatment with factor VIII

- More serious injuries and bleeds
  — These include:

  Any hard blow on the head, especially if the child is dazed

  Any injury to the face, mouth or neck – danger signs are any difficulty in swallowing or breathing

  Abdominal injuries or any unexplained abdominal pain

  Lacerations that are severe enough to need stitching

  — If these occur, the child should be transferred to the haemophilia centre by the quickest means available and the parents and haematologist informed

HYDROCEPHALUS

- Can be congenital or acquired
- Acquired secondary to meningitis, intracranial haemorrhage, severe head injury or brain tumours

Diagnosis
- Congenital
  — May be diagnosed on antenatal ultrasounds
- Acquired
  — Intraventricular haemorrhage in pre-term infants on cranial ultrasound
  — Head injuries – accidents or non-accidental injury
  — Tumours on CT scan

Shunts
- CSF is diverted from the lateral ventricles to the abdominal cavity usually via a valve (i.e. Spitz–Holtzer). Blocked shunts will result in 'bulging' of the diaphragms on these valves or poor refilling. This should be checked only by a neurosurgical team

Possible symptoms of shunt malformation
- In all children
  — Vomiting
  — Irritability
  — Lethargy
  — Seizures
  — Swelling or redness along shunt tract
- In babies
  — Above or bulging fontanelle, change in appetite and sunsetting eyes

Arrange for urgent referral.

DRUG AND SOLVENT ABUSE IN SCHOOL CHILDREN

- Common – as many as 20% of 11–16 year olds have used solvents or illegal drugs at least once
- Not confined to any particular group
- Most involvement is temporary/casual
- Reasons for involvement:
  — Peer pressure
  — Experimentation and kicks
  — To boost self-esteem
- A minority progress to multiple drug use, chronic use, and addiction (usually an extension of delinquent behaviour associated with other problems)
- Likelihood of experimentation increases with age; male:female 3:2
- Chronic drug users are more likely to come from families where adults are dependent on drugs, e.g. alcohol, tranquillizers
- Multiple drug use may be associated with:
  — Early use of tobacco and alcohol
  — Mixing with older children
  — Increased early sexual experience
- The following may be associated with substance abuse:
  — Persistent truancy
  — Behaviour/personality changes, e.g. unusually withdrawn, uncharacteristic outbursts, labile mood
  — Loss of interest in appearance, school work, hobbies or sport
  — Loss of appetite
  — Bouts of lethargy, drowsiness, unsteady gait
  — Unexplained deterioration in school progress
  — Furtive behaviour, often associated with stealing
  — Unusual stains or smells on body or clothing

General effects
- Most amplify mood, e.g. depression, anxiety, aggression
- Many alter mood giving exhilaration, confidence
- Many alter perceptions, e.g. visual, auditory
- Most weaken personal and social inhibitions
- Most impair reaction time, control and concentration
- Individual response to drugs varies
- Illegal drugs are unpredictable in strength and quality
- Combining drugs increases the effects and the risks, e.g. alcohol plus solvents

Risks
Death
- Uncommon
- Most often due to accidents associated with impaired physical and mental functioning

- Can occur due to inhalation of vomit in unconscious state
- Can be due to method of administration, e.g. asphyxia in solvent abuse
- Can be due to direct toxic effect of drug (idiosyncratic and unpredictable)

Chronic drug use resulting in:
- Deterioration in social relations
- Deterioration in mental functioning
- Deterioration in diet and health
- Dependence
  — Psychological (more common)
  — Physical (rarer) alcohol, nicotine, opiates, sedatives

Injection use
- Hepatitis B
- Septicaemia
- HIV, AIDS

Specific drugs – legal
Alcohol
- Often implicated in antisocial and criminal behaviour
- 90% of girls and 95% of boys of 13 years have tried alcohol
- 33% of these are regular drinkers (most often small amounts in own home)
- Heavy drinkers often proceed to abuse multiple drugs
- Trend towards earlier drinking and consuming stronger sources of alcohol such as spirits and strong lager

Nicotine
- Drug most responsible for widespread health damage (respiratory and cardiovascular)
- Will kill one quarter of its regular users
- 10% of 11–15 year olds smoke regularly
- Almost as many girls as boys smoke
- Smoking has increased from 1992–94 from 13% to 18% of 14–15 year olds

Solvents
- Similar effects to alcohol but rapid onset
- Age range 7–18, prevalence 10%, male:female 3:1
- Usually a group activity
- 2% go on to become regular abusers – may be a lone activity; associated with social deprivation
- Deaths from solvent abuse:
  — 90% are boys aged 11–17
  — More young people die from solvent abuse than 'hard drugs'
  — Approximately 2 per week in UK
  — More than 75% deaths are sudden
  — 53% caused by heart failure
  — 10% caused by suffocation (in plastic bags)

- Substances used
  - Glues
  - Cleaning fluids
  - Paint thinners
  - Aerosols
  - Butane
- Methods used
  - Sniffed or swallowed directly from container – bottles, tubes, pens, plastic bag (danger of asphyxia)
  - Onto rag or clothing and sniffed, sucked or chewed
  - Spraying directly into mouth, e.g. butane (danger of laryngeal spasm/oedema and death)
- Effects:
  - Rapid onset and recovery with little hangover
  - Light-headedness, dizziness, euphoria, hallucinations drowsiness
  - Psychological dependence, fatigue, depression, liver and kidney damage, lead poisoning if sniffing leaded petrol, long-term heavy use may cause significant brain impairment
  - 30–50% of trips can be frightening
- Diagnosis
  - Smell on breath lasts 24 hours
  - Glue on clothes or skin
  - 'Glue sniffers' rash' around mouth a late sign of prolonged use
- Management
  - Acute coma management. (In mouth to mouth resuscitation, risk of intoxication of resuscitator)
  - History: what? how? how often? why?
  - Advise child on risks: lone sniffing, dangerous administration practices
  - Check urea and electrolytes and liver function tests
  - This excludes damage but also emphasises potential dangers
  - Reassure parents that damage is infrequent and addiction rare
  - Family therapy for chronic users

Specific drugs – illegal

Cannabis (dope, grass, hash, weed, pot, joint – many others)
- Causes disorientation, relaxation, heightened awareness, decrease in concentration and dexterity; lasts several hours
- Commonest used illegal drug – 13–28% 15+ year olds have tried it
- Smoked with tobacco or on its own in pipe, or ingested
- Recent evidence suggests there may be long-term health risks

Cocaine (coke, snow, charlie)
- Powerful stimulant giving exhilaration, euphoria, reduced need to sleep, indifference to pain and hunger and often panic
- Usually sniffed through a tube (snorting), licked from finger (dabbing) or placed in rectum. Sometimes dissolved and injected

- Peak effect 15–40 minutes and rapidly wears off leaving insomnia, fatigue and depression
- Long-term problems – anxiety, insomnia, weight loss, exhaustion, paranoia

Crack cocaine (rock, wash, base)
- Similar effects to cocaine, more intense euphoria
- Smoked in cigarette or pipe or burnt on foil and inhaled
- Tolerance, agitation and paranoia may occur

Heroin (smack, H, Harry, skag, junk) and other opiates
- Causes euphoria, contentment and warmth with little depression in moderate doses; effects immediate and can last several hours
- Sedation and coma in excessive dosage
- Dissolved and injected, smoked on tin foil (chasing the dragon) or sniffed
- Tolerance and physical dependence – withdrawal symptoms start after 8–24 hours and generally fade in 7–10 days
- There may be adulterants in preparation

Amphetamines (speed, whizz, billy, sulphate, dexies, pink champagne)
- Give energy, confidence and exhilaration, but also irritability, panic or psychosis; can last 3–4 hours
- Usually sniffed through a tube (snorting), licked from finger (dabbing). Sometimes dissolved and injected
- Can cause tolerance, anorexia, amenorrhoea or infertility

Ecstasy (MDMA, adam, E, XTC, white doves, lone doves, disco burgers)
- Feelings of well being, heightened awareness, panic; effects last 2–8 hours
- Tablets or capsules swallowed
- May cause personality change, depression, anxiety

LSD (acid, trips, tabs)
- Causes a prolonged 'trip' (a variable unpredictable experience ranging from ecstasy to disorientation and panic); peak effect 2–3 hours, fading after 12 hours
- Swallowed, sniffed or injected
- Death due to suicide rare. May have long-term disorientation or paranoia

Magic mushrooms (liberty cap, psilocybe)
- Causes euphoria, hallucinatory effects, anxiety; may last 9–12 hours
- Eaten fresh or dried, or made into tea or soup
- Potential for mistakenly eating poisonous varieties

Barbiturates (barbs, sleepers, downers, yellow jackets, rainbow)
- Causes relaxation, sleepiness, slurred speech; lasts 3–6 hours
- Tablets or capsules swallowed
- Can cause chronic fatigue, memory loss, depression, insomnia

Tranquillizers – benzodiazepines (tranx, benzos, jellies, blobs)
- Causes relaxation, drowsiness; lasts 8–10 hours, effects can be cumulative
- Tablets or capsules swallowed, temazepam gel may be injected
- Highly addictive in long-term use

Nitrites (poppers, snappers, liquid gold, rush, locker room)
- Muscle relaxant, enhances sexual sensations, vasodilatation
- Liquid in glass bottle or capsule sniffed or left open in room, effects last up to 5 minutes
- Can cause headaches, vomiting. may be carcinogenic. Dangerous in people with cardiovascular problems

Help and information
- Information (leaflets and videos) may be obtained from local health education departments
- Help for individuals may be obtained from drug addiction units
- Police liaison may also be most useful
- Institute for the Study of Drug Dependence (ISDD) – information on drugs
  > 1 Hatton Place
  > London
  > EC1N 8ND
  > Tel: 0171 803 4720
- The Standing Conference on Drug Abuse (SCODA) – information on local services
  > 1–4 Hatton Place
  > London
  > EC1N 8ND
  > Tel: 0171 928 9500
- Release – 24-hour drug line
  > Tel: 0171 603 8654

ALCOHOL

- There are many similarities between smoking and alcohol consumption with overlap of risk factors contributing to teenage alcohol intake
- Complete prohibition of teenage alcohol consumption is difficult but *sensible* drinking should be promoted
- Safe limits – not assessed for teenagers. 14 units/week for adult women and 21 units/week for adult men. One unit = $\frac{1}{2}$ pint beer/lager or one measure of whiskey

Dangers of acute alcohol intoxication

Medical
- Hypoglycaemia
- Aspiration of vomit

- Irregular menstrual periods with chronic alcohol abuse
- Hangover

Social
- Decreased social inhibition with increased sexual activity, particularly unprotected sex
- Association with violence, drink driving (illegal as under 16!), accidents and smoking
- Absenteeism from school

Tackling the problem

Individuals during consultation
- Elicit history. Identify social factors which manifest as 'alcoholism', i.e. child abuse, parental alcoholism, dysfunctional family. These need addressing first:
- Try introducing 'alcohol-free days'
- Don't use alcohol to cope with emotional problems
- Don't drink alone
- If drinking with friends – intersperse alcohol with non-alcoholic or low-alcohol drinks
- Don't take drugs when drinking
- Don't drink on an empty stomach
- Put your glass down between sips and try to pace drinking so you become one of the slower drinkers in company; sip, don't gulp
- If drinking spirits always dilute them
- Emphasise cost

Health promotion
- Similar principle to smoking when advocating 'sensible drinking'
- Need support for teenagers who drink excessively. Consider referral to local child psychiatrists or establish 'support group' with help from psychiatrists/school nurses

SMOKING

- Smoking is the largest cause of preventable deaths (adults and children), accounting for 5 times the mortality of all the other avoidable deaths put together (road accidents, suicide, drugs, etc.). Tobacco smoke contains thousands of chemicals, of which 60 are known or suspected carcinogens

Smoking-related illness (adults)
- Lung cancer – 80% associated with smoking
- Causal associations with mouth, pharyngeal, larynx, oesophageal, bladder, pancreas, renal and cervical cancers
- Cardiovascular disease
    — Up to 18% of CHD disease associated with smoking
    — Up to 11% of smoke deaths
- Chronic bronchitis – 80% associated with smoking

- Sexual health
  — May affect fertility
  — Increased fetal and perinatal mortality by one-third
  — Increased risk of pre-term delivery (twice as common in smokers)

Passive smoking
- Increased incidence of:
  — Respiratory illness from birth to 3 years, especially bronchiolitis and pneumonia
  — Chronic otitis media
  — Acute exacerbation of asthma in known asthmatics and implicated as a risk factor in the development of asthma
  — Cot death
  — Small increase in later lung cancer

Prevalence
- 28% of adults in England are regular smokers, with a gradual decline in prevalence (1992 CHS data)
- Teenagers, though, are smoking more over time, with 23% of 15 year olds smoking at least one cigarette a week. 70% of all 16 year olds would have tried smoking at one stage too

Health promotion among parents – see 'Health Promotion' section
- Most are aware of the dangers (88% of public aware of link with lung cancer and 74% with heart disease). 'Education' alone does not alter lifestyle

Health promotion in teenagers
- When to start – debatable, but early experimentation starts at 9–11 years with a sudden escalation in prevalence from 12–13 years till 16 years

What sort of programme?
- Crucial to understand why they smoke before embarking on programme
- Multi-factorial
  — Poor self-esteem
  — Peer group pressure – the need to conform particularly if low self-esteem
  — Role models – both parental and teachers together with TV personalities
  — Advertising
  — Cost of cigarettes

There are other factors which influence individuals.

How
- Multi-disciplinary – including teachers and school nurses
- Health education needs to address issues of importance to

teenagers, i.e. bad breath and cost as opposed to 'health risks when they are old' which are less powerful images. Useful to get their feedback and empower them to educate themselves

- Health education needs to be supported by programmes which address those factors above (i.e. self-esteem and peer group pressure)
- Support measures to limit availability, i.e. cost. It is illegal to sell cigarettes to under 16 years olds yet the majority of them obtain cigarettes from corner shops/newsagents, etc.

SEX EDUCATION

- By the age of 16, 18.7% of females and 27.6% of males have engaged in sexual intercourse. This is significant as:
    - Risk of sexually transmitted disease, i.e. HIV
    - Teenage pregnancy with increased maternal and fetal physiological risk factors
    - Correlation between cervical cancer and early sexual intercourse

Adolescents establish their views from parental, peer and media influences. Formal sex education within schools emphasise 'lifeskills' – the ability to cope with and establish healthy relationships. This is usually by encouraging individuals to identify with real situations and experiences together with clarifying their own attitudes and values. There is less emphasis upon didactic lectures to improve education.

- This adolescent-centred approach encourages individuals to examine their own values and practices
- Health professionals can be involved in:
    - School programmes as an integral member, i.e. school nurse/doctor discussing contraception
    - Linked to school nurse health appraisal
    - Opportunistic consultations
        Advice on the 'morning after pill' following unprotected intercourse
        Contraceptive advice
        Presentation with other medical problems, i.e. abdominal pain but really concerned about sexual health
    - Being used as an alternative information source (to above) when discussing general issues or behaviour problems. This is especially relevant to children with learning and physical disability

Approach
- Group work – usually organized by school
- Individual – support/advice dependent on history
- Use similar principles to other aspects of health promotion
    - Identify concerns about self-esteem/peer pressure

- — Sensitively explore knowledge (or lack) of contraception – most claim awareness
- — Get the adolescent to identify situations which 'could lead too far', i.e. inhibitions lowered by alcohol, saying 'no' if petting/physical contact becomes uncomfortable
- Establish what emotional support network the adolescent depends upon. The quality of the friendships within the network is more important than the quantity of friends. The lack of quality support increases peer pressure, especially in someone of low self-esteem. This increases the risk of the adolescent compromizing their own values or expectations of sexual relationships
- Spend time *listening*. Many need more than one session
- Be aware of your own limitations. You may appear pejorative if the consultations contradicts your personal morality. It is *not* an admission of failure to refer the adolescent to a colleague
- Ensure confidentiality (unless involving sexual abuse)

POISONING

- Remember that poisoning can be an indication of family disruption

Drugs
- Less common since the introduction of child-resistant containers, but they are not child proof

Aspirin
- Acidosis leading to hyperventilation
- Coma is late

Paracetamol
- No immediate problems, but hepatic and renal damage can be serious and cause death

Tricyclics
- May have been prescribed for an older sibling's enuresis
- Causes cardiac arrhythmias and coma
- Commonest cause of death from poisoning in children

Iron
- Often prescribed for pregnant mothers
- Early symptoms: nausea, vomiting, haematemesis
- Late: encephalopathy and circulatory collapse
- Later: liver necrosis

Benzodiazepines
- Cause general sedation
- Transfer to hospital

Management
- Give activated charcoal as soon as possible to reduce absorption

- Salt should never be given

- Transfer to casualty if there is any possibility that a dangerous amount has been taken
- Always send a sample for identification

Household products

Bleach
- Irritate mouth and oesophagus and may cause stricture

Caustic soda
- Rarely enough ingested to cause systemic effects

Turpentine
- May be inhaled and cause chemical pneumonia

Paraffin
- CNS problems if taken in large quantities

Management

- *Do not induce vomiting* because of the risk of repeat trauma to the oesophagus and inhalation
- Dilute in stomach with drinks (preferably milk) or bind with activated charcoal
- Transfer to hospital if concern about amount ingested

Plants, berries etc.

- These rarely cause serious problems
- Identify product if possible
- Induce vomiting and transfer to hospital if uncertain about how dangerous it might be

Alcohol

- In children, causes dangerous hypoglycaemia
- Transfer to hospital unless certain that a minimal amount has been taken

Follow-up

- Following an episode of ingestion of a potentially dangerous substance, it is valuable to check upon safety at home
  — Are drugs locked away always?
  — Are household products stored out of reach?
  — Are containers well labelled?
  — Are garage contents safe?

Useful telephone numbers

- Poisons information centres:

Belfast	01232–240503
Birmingham	0121–554 3801
Cardiff	01222–709901
Dublin	379964 or Dublin 379966
Edinburgh	0131–229 2477
Leeds	0113–243 0715 or 0113–292 3547
London	0171–635 9191 or 0171–955 5095
Newcastle	0191–232 5131

DENTAL SERVICES

Dental caries

Bacteria + carbohydrate $\rightarrow$ acid $\rightarrow$ decalcification $\rightarrow$ secondary bacterial invasion

Caused by:
- Debris on teeth – especially carbohydrate
- Poor dental hygiene
- Dietary sugar
  - Sweets
  - Sugars in drinks (and medicines)
- Early decay can be caused by sweetened dummies, or continual drink bottle in mouth

Prevention
- Balanced diet
- Clean teeth twice daily (performed/supervised by parent until 7 years old)
- Regular dental examination every 6 months
- An adequate intake of fluoride will protect against dental decay
  - Supplements as tablets or drops are required if the level in drinking water is low
  - Consult the district dental officer about local levels
- The doctor, health visitors and community nurses can reinforce the need for good dental care
- The care of the teeth may be a useful indicator of care overall
- In some children poor teeth is associated with poor general nutrition

Services
- General dental practitioner
- Secondary hospital services
- Community dental services

Children should be registered and seen by the dentist as early as possible.
- By age 3 the child should be used to the dentist
- Parents should be encouraged to take their child to their own family dentist or to the local community dentist
- The community dental service may offer the following services for children (local services vary):
  - Annual dental screening for all children in school
  - Clinics in some local health centres to provide treatment and advice
  - Mobile clinics that can visit special schools and centres
  - A domiciliary service
  - Priority preventive counselling for pre-school children with learning difficulties

— Dental health education through schools, clubs, ante-natal groups etc.

Conditions of importance to the dentist
- The dentist should be informed about the following medical problems, which:
    - Require special precautions, e.g. bleeding disorders, congenital heart disease
    - Increase general anaesthetic risk, e.g. asthma, epilepsy
    - Increase risk of dental disease, e.g. immune incompetence
    - May be worsened by dental disease, e.g. diabetes
    - Make dental care more difficult, e.g. learning difficulty, cerebral palsy
    - Put the dentist at risk, e.g. hepatitis B, HIV

ANAEMIA

Identification
- Skin pallor unreliable except for severe anaemia
- Inspection of the tarsal conjunctiva for pallor
- Pallor of the pinnae may give a clue
- Blue sclera may be found in iron deficiency
- General lack of energy/ill health
- Tachycardia
- Flow murmur

Children at higher risk of anaemia
- Children from deprived families or where there are nutritional problems, e.g. due to late weaning
- Preterm infants due to lack of iron stores
- Greek and Asian children due to thalassaemia
- African and West Indian children due to sickle-cell disease

If the child is clinically anaemic ask the following:
- Is there bleeding?
- Is it nutritional?
- Is there haemolysis?
- Is there an underlying cause – chronic renal disease, collagen/vascular, chronic infection; TB?

- Commonest problems seen in the community are due to iron deficiency and haemoglobinopathy

If anaemia suspected ask for:
- Full blood count
- Film
- Haemoglobin electrophoresis if appropriate
- Ferritin

- Consider calcium, phosphate, alkaline phosphatase if nutritional anaemia suspected as this may co-exist with other deficiencies, e.g. vitamin D

Interpretation of results

Iron deficiency
- Microcytic, hypochromic film diagnostic
- Low ferritin

Thalassaemia
- Target cells
- Raised level of HbA2 on electrophoresis (normally 1–3%; 3–6% in thalassaemia trait)

Sickle-cell anaemia
- Sickle-cells seen in film under reduced oxygen tension
- Electrophoresis HbS

Iron-deficiency anaemia

- Commonest in the older pre-school child after weaning onto a diet with inadequate iron content, when introduction of solids is late or when the child is drinking excess milk or orange squash
- Up to 40% of children in some inner-city areas are iron deficient
- Iron deficiency also causes:
  - Developmental delay
  - Increased susceptibility to infection
  - Poor appetite, pica
  - Behavioural difficulties
- Prevention
  - Wean onto foods with a high iron content
  - Fortified cereals – iron in breakfast cereals is an underrated source
  - Bread
  - Eggs
  - Fish
  - Meat
  - Pulses (lentils, peas, baked beans)
  - The iron in green vegetables is not well absorbed
  - Iron fortified 'follow-on' milks are not superior to a good weaning diet
- Management
  - Look for iron deficiency in other family members
  - Look for other dietary deficiencies – vitamin D deficiency commonly co-exists
  - Dietary management is preferable in children with mild/moderate anaemia (Hb over 9 g)
  - Dietary management will also correct other deficiencies
  - Vitamin C, given as fresh fruit or fruit juice, will enhance the absorption of iron

- Dietary advice, in order to be successful, may need to be combined with measures to increase income (benefits) or regulate its expenditure (budgeting)
- A general practice based intervention educational programme reduced iron deficiency from 25 to 8%
- If anaemia is severe (Hb less than 9 g) or it is unlikely that dietary advice can or will be followed, then an oral iron preparation is needed
- Warn of the dangers of accidental ingestion of iron and advise on storage
- Follow-up
  - Repeat haemoglobin and ferritin levels after 3 months to ensure adequacy of treatment and response
  - If inadequate response, consider
    Poor compliance
    Blood loss
  - Continued nutritional surveillance as problems often recur

Sickle-cell anaemia
- Antenatal diagnosis is available by chorionic villous biopsy
- Diagnosis from cord blood in areas of high incidence facilitates rapid action by parents when serious complications occur, where prior appropriate counselling has been given
- Heterozygotes with up to 35% of HbS are asymptomatic and are not anaemic
  - They require advice on anaesthesia, and air travel as sickling may occur under hypoxic conditions (dentist should be informed)
  - They may require genetic counselling
- Homozygotes have 80–95% HbS
  - They may present with:
    Painful crises, due to infarction
    Aplastic crises (due to parvovirus infection)
    Megaloblastic crises due to folate deficiency (very rare)
    Haemolytic crises
    Splenic sequestration (may require splenectomy if repeated); common cause of death
    Hepatic crises due to obstructive jaundice
    Neurological complications (strokes) which are an indication for management by transfusion to suppress bone marrow production of sickle haemoglobin
    Other clinical problems include ulceration around the ankles, infection with *Salmonella*, which may cause osteomyelitis, and persistent signs of pneumonia, probably due to infarction
  - Enuresis due to inability to concentrate urine is a problem
    Dryness is eventually achieved

— Growth may be impaired due to delay in puberty, but catch-up growth can be expected
— School attainment may be impaired due to loss of schooling or cerebral sickling
  Consider transfusion therapy
— They require
  Folic acid supplements
  Prompt treatment of infections
  Penicillin prophylaxis throughout childhood to prevent pneumococcal infection – a pneumococcal vaccine (Pneumovax) is also available
  Transfusion if neurological complications have occurred (suppresses formation of own red cells)
  Genetic counselling
  In general, normal school and curriculum (teachers need careful explanation and advice on obtaining medical help if crises occur)
— School leavers will need advice as exercise tolerance may be limited by anaemia, bone pain or leg ulcers

Thalassaemia

- Found in children originating from countries around the Mediterranean, most commonly Turkey and Greece, and also from Middle and Far East and Africa
- Children with beta-thalassaemia major
  — Severe anaemia
  — Gross enlargement of liver and spleen
  — Require regular transfusion
  — Need desferrioxamine to delay onset of haemosiderosis
  — Families require genetic counselling
  — Few survive into middle life
- Children with thalassaemia trait
  — Are mildly anaemic (Hb 10–12 g/dl)
  — Do not require treatment
  — Must not be given iron as this may lead to haemosiderosis
  — Need genetic counselling

5. CHARTS AND TABLES

I DEVELOPMENT 0–5

The boxes corresponding to the child's chronological age are filled in (horizontal axis) against the age-related developmental items on the left. One box must be filled in for each item achieved.

90% of children will complete items above the black line. Those 10% scoring below the line should be referred or re-assessed within a month.

Allowances must be made for prematurity when filling out these charts.

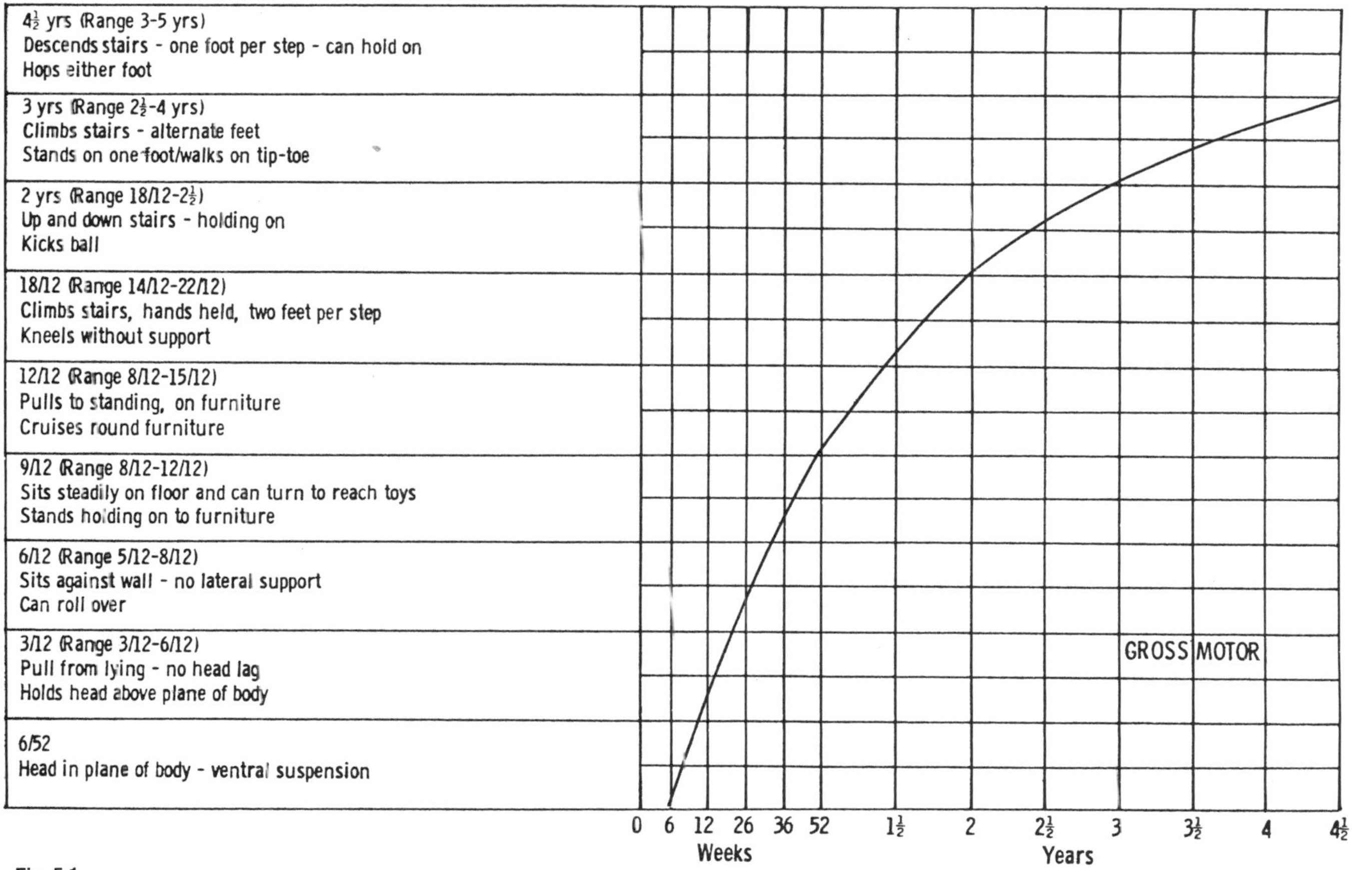
4½ yrs (Range 3-5 yrs)
Descends stairs - one foot per step - can hold on
Hops either foot
3 yrs (Range 2½-4 yrs)
Climbs stairs - alternate feet
Stands on one foot/walks on tip-toe
2 yrs (Range 18/12-2½)
Up and down stairs - holding on
Kicks ball
18/12 (Range 14/12-22/12)
Climbs stairs, hands held, two feet per step
Kneels without support
12/12 (Range 8/12-15/12)
Pulls to standing, on furniture
Cruises round furniture
9/12 (Range 8/12-12/12)
Sits steadily on floor and can turn to reach toys
Stands holding on to furniture
6/12 (Range 5/12-8/12)
Sits against wall - no lateral support
Can roll over
3/12 (Range 3/12-6/12)
Pull from lying - no head lag
Holds head above plane of body
6/52
Head in plane of body - ventral suspension
GROSS MOTOR
0 6 12 26 36 52
Weeks
1½ 2 2½ 3 3½ 4 4½
Years

Fig. 5.1

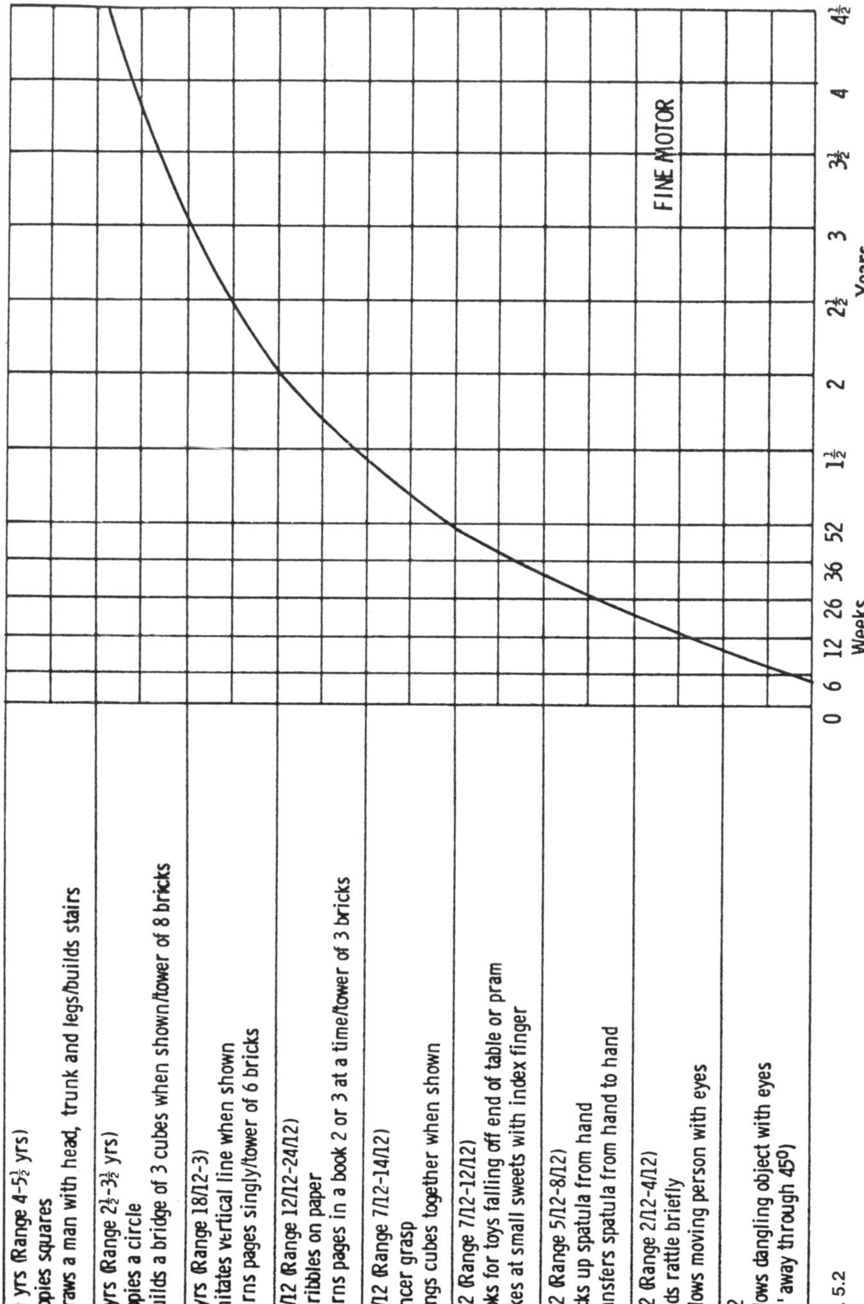

FINE MOTOR

4½ yrs (Range 4-5½ yrs)
Copies squares
Draws a man with head, trunk and legs/builds stairs

3 yrs (Range 2½-3½ yrs)
Copies a circle
Builds a bridge of 3 cubes when shown/tower of 8 bricks

2 yrs (Range 18/12-3)
Imitates vertical line when shown
Turns pages singly/tower of 6 bricks

18/12 (Range 12/12-24/12)
Scribbles on paper
Turns pages in a book 2 or 3 at a time/tower of 3 bricks

12/12 (Range 7/12-14/12)
Pincer grasp
Bangs cubes together when shown

9/12 (Range 7/12-12/12)
Looks for toys falling off end of table or pram
Pokes at small sweets with index finger

6/12 (Range 5/12-8/12)
Picks up spatula from hand
Transfers spatula from hand to hand

3/12 (Range 2/12-4/12)
Holds rattle briefly
Follows moving person with eyes

6/52
Follows dangling object with eyes
(12" away through 45°)

0 6 12 26 36 52 1½ 2 2½ 3 3½ 4 4½
Weeks   Years

Fig. 5.2

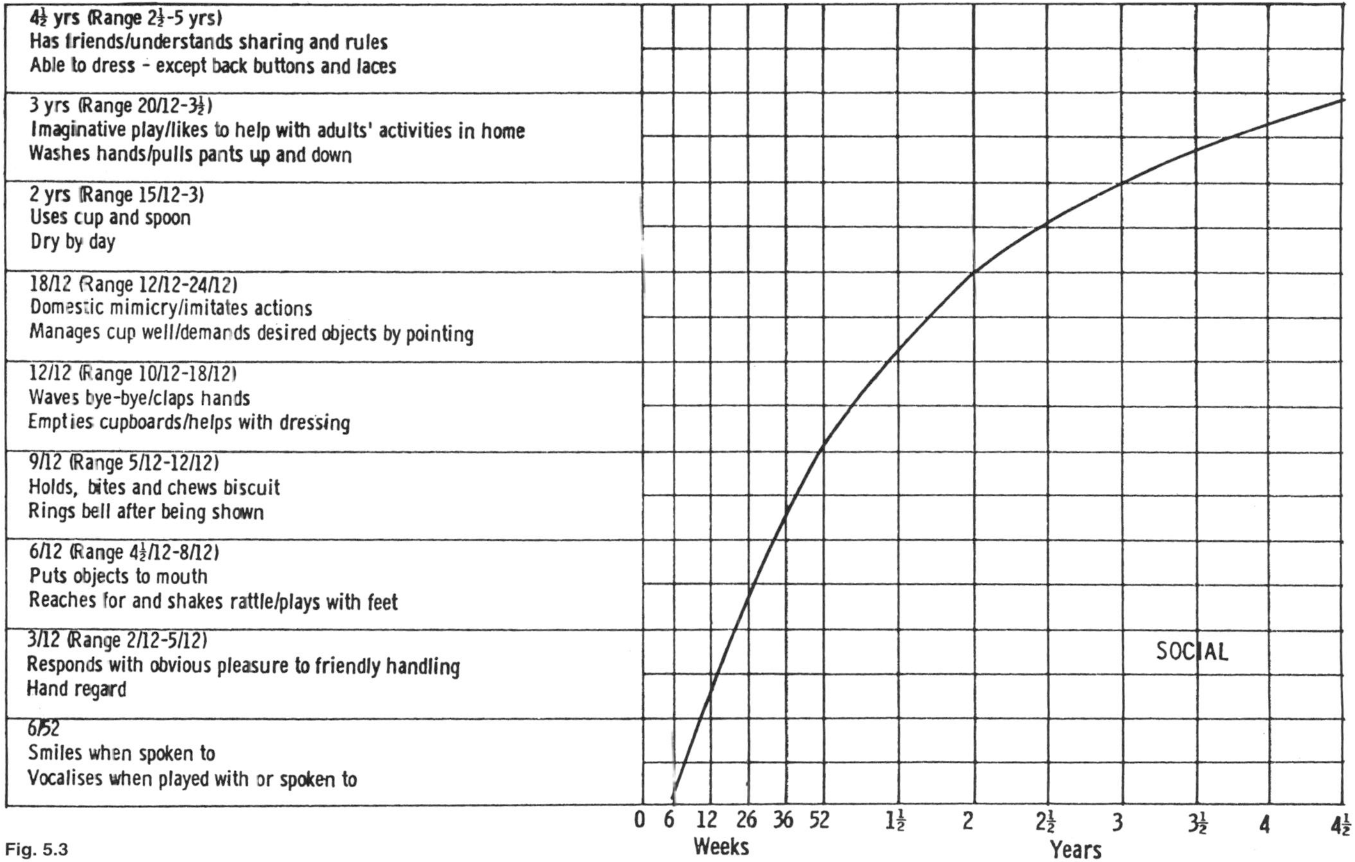
4½ yrs (Range 2½-5 yrs)
Has friends/understands sharing and rules
Able to dress - except back buttons and laces
3 yrs (Range 20/12-3½)
Imaginative play/likes to help with adults' activities in home
Washes hands/pulls pants up and down
2 yrs (Range 15/12-3)
Uses cup and spoon
Dry by day
18/12 (Range 12/12-24/12)
Domestic mimicry/imitates actions
Manages cup well/demands desired objects by pointing
12/12 (Range 10/12-18/12)
Waves bye-bye/claps hands
Empties cupboards/helps with dressing
9/12 (Range 5/12-12/12)
Holds, bites and chews biscuit
Rings bell after being shown
6/12 (Range 4½/12-8/12)
Puts objects to mouth
Reaches for and shakes rattle/plays with feet
3/12 (Range 2/12-5/12)
Responds with obvious pleasure to friendly handling
Hand regard
6/52
Smiles when spoken to
Vocalises when played with or spoken to
SOCIAL
0 6 12 26 36 52
Weeks
1½ 2 2½ 3 3½ 4 4½
Years

Fig. 5.3

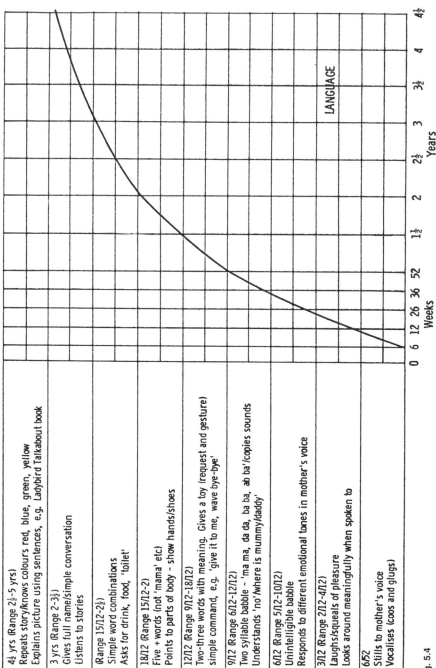

Fig. 5.4

4½ yrs (Range 2½-5 yrs)
Repeats story/knows colours red, blue, green, yellow
Explains picture using sentences, e.g. Ladybird Talkabout book

3 yrs (Range 2-3½)
Gives full name/simple conversation
Listens to stories

(Range 15/12-2½)
Simple word combinations
Asks for drink, food, 'toilet'

18/12 (Range 15/12-2)
Five + words (not 'mama' etc)
Points to parts of body – show hands/shoes

12/12 (Range 9/12-18/12)
Two-three words with meaning. Gives a toy (request and gesture)
simple command, e.g. 'give it to me, wave bye-bye'

9/12 (Range 6/12-12/12)
Two syllable babble – 'ma ma, da da, ba ba, ab ba'/copies sounds
Understands 'no'/where is mummy/daddy'

6/12 (Range 5/12-10/12)
Unintelligible babble
Responds to different emotional tones in mother's voice

3/12 (Range 2/12-4/12)
Laughs/squeals of pleasure
Looks around meaningfully when spoken to

6/52
Stills to mother's voice
Vocalises (coos and glugs)

LANGUAGE

0 6 12 26 36 52   1½   2   2½   3   3½   4   4½
      Weeks   Years

II GROWTH CHARTS

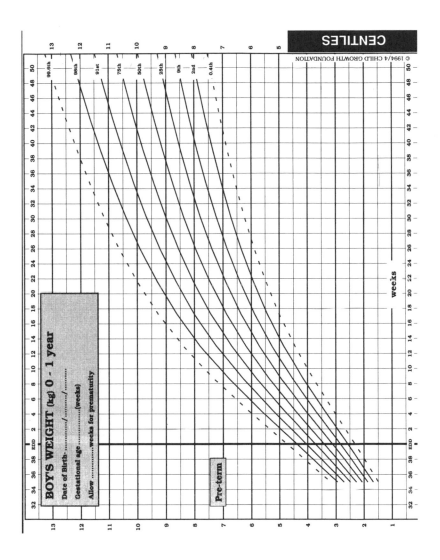

Fig. 5.5 Boy's weight 0–1 year

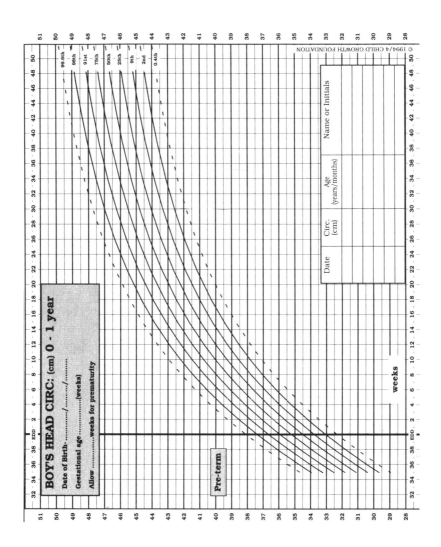

Fig. 5.6 Boy's head circ 0–1 year

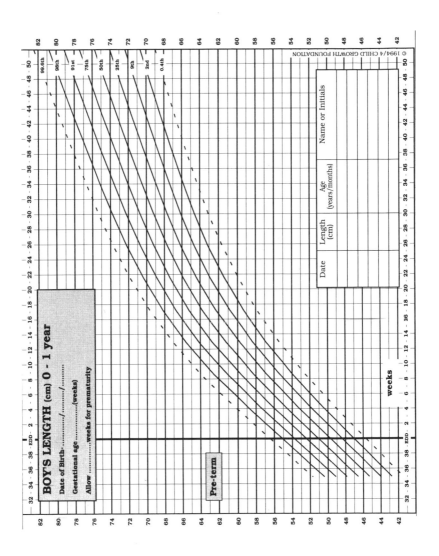

Fig. 5.7 Boy's length 0–1 year

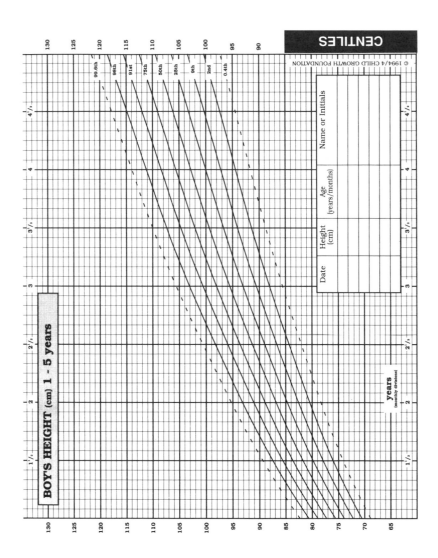

Fig. 5.8 Boy's height 1–5 years

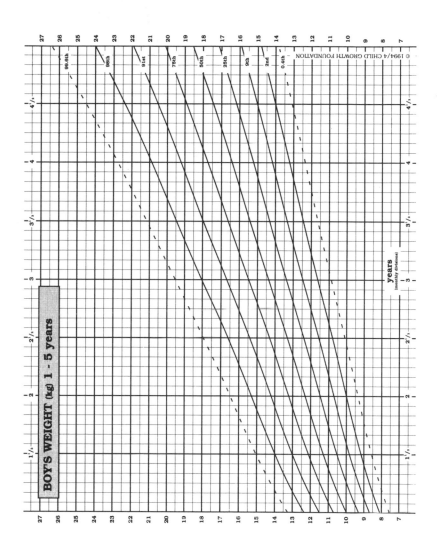

Fig. 5.9 Boy's weight 1–5 years

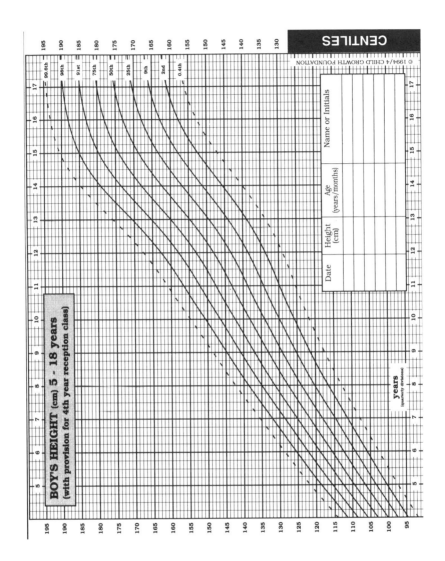

Fig. 5.10 Boy's height 5–18 years

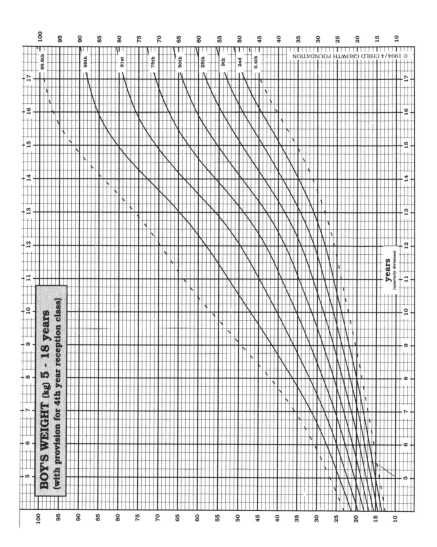

Fig. 5.11 Boy's weight 5–18 years

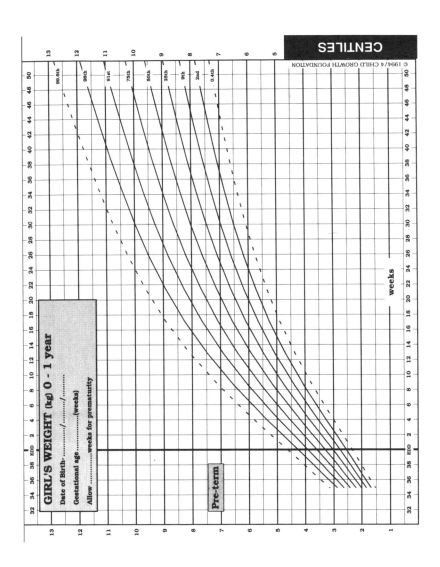

Fig. 5.12 Girl's weight 0–1 year

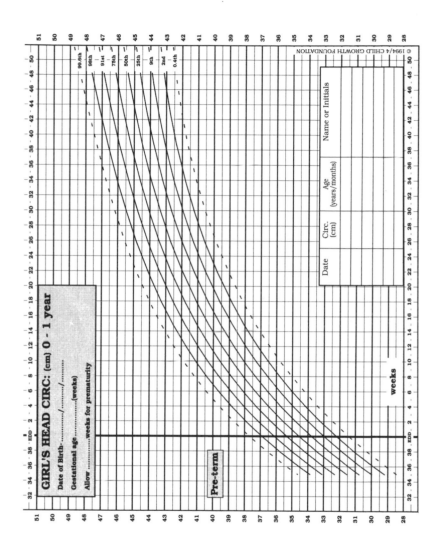

Fig. 5.13 Girl's head circ 0–1 year

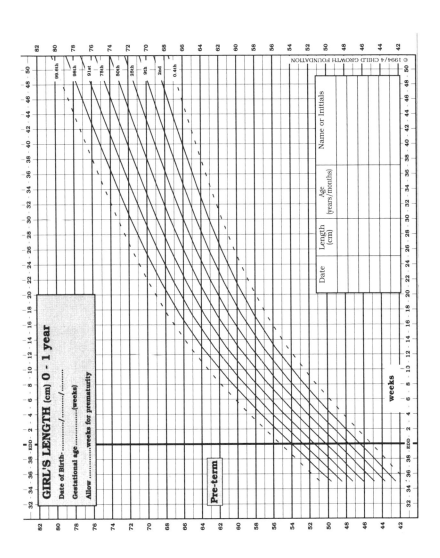

Fig. 5.14 Girl's length 0–1 year

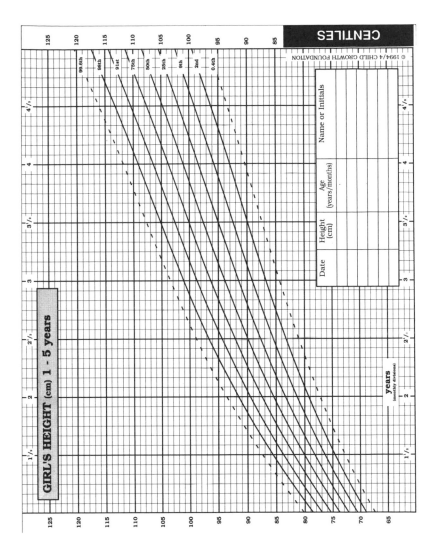

Fig. 5.15 Girl's height 1–5 years

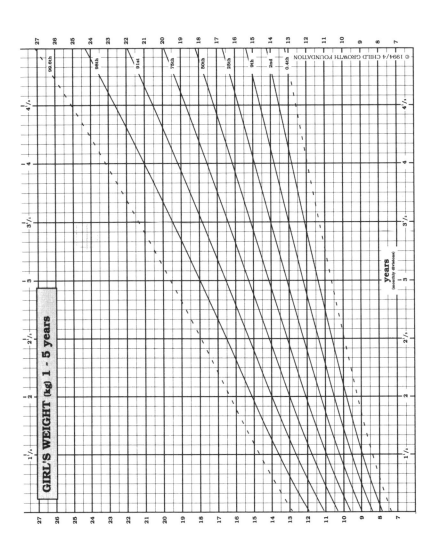

Fig. 5.16 Girl's weight 1–5 years

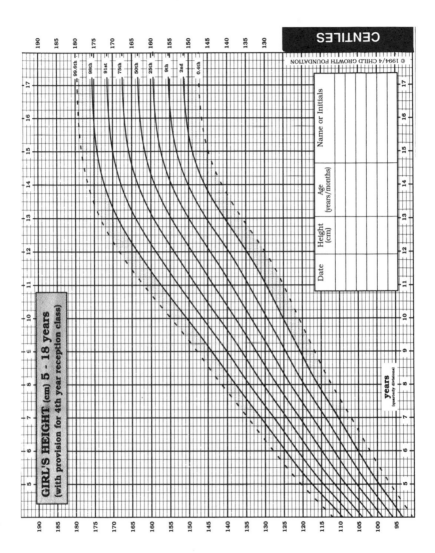

Fig. 5.17 Girl's height 5–18 years

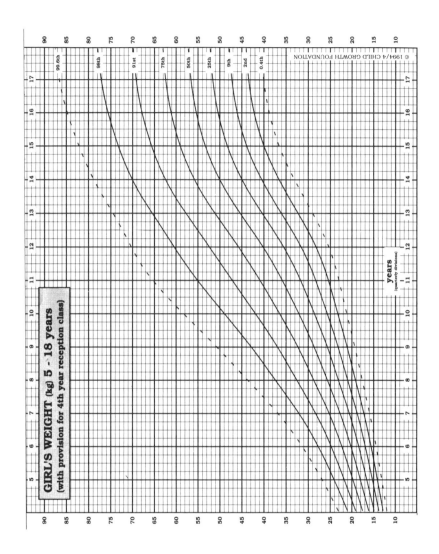

Fig. 5.18 Girl's weight 5–18 years

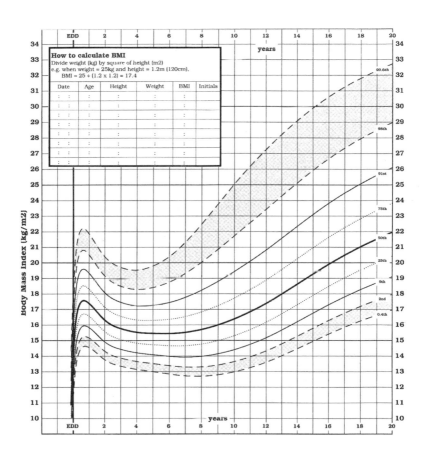

Fig. 5.19 Body mass index chart – boys

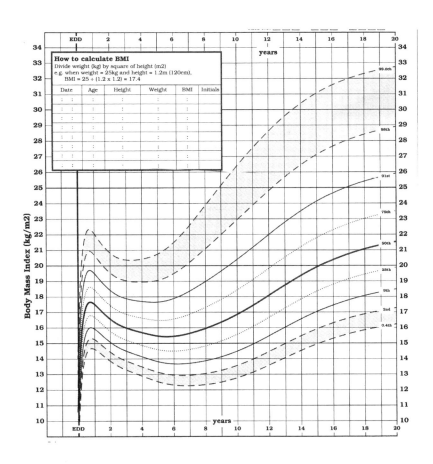

How to calculate BMI
Divide weight (kg) by square of height (m2)
e.g. when weight = 25kg and height = 1.2m (120cm),
BMI = 25 ÷ (1.2 x 1.2) = 17.4

Date	Age	Height	Weight	BMI	Initials
: :	:	:	:	:	:
: :	:	:	:	:	:
: :	:	:	:	:	:
: :	:	:	:	:	:
: :	:	:	:	:	:
: :	:	:	:	:	:
: :	:	:	:	:	:

Fig. 5.20 Body mass index chart – girls

III MISCELLANEOUS CHARTS

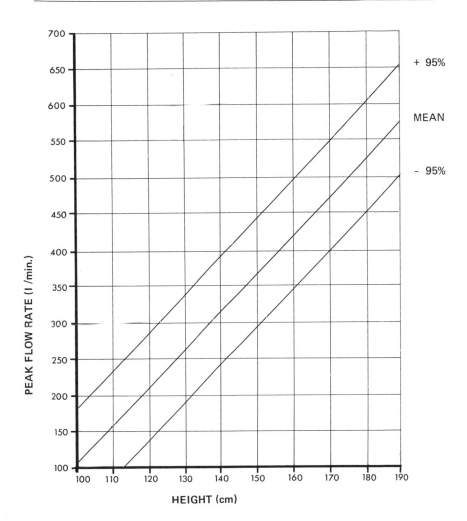

Fig. 5.21 Peak flow

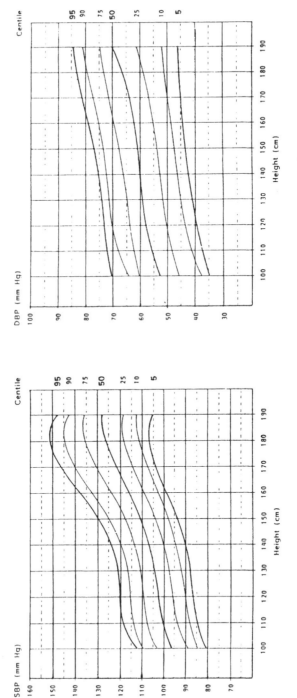

Fig. 5.22 Height-specific blood pressure percentiles – boys

Fig. 5.23 Height-specific blood pressure percentiles – girls

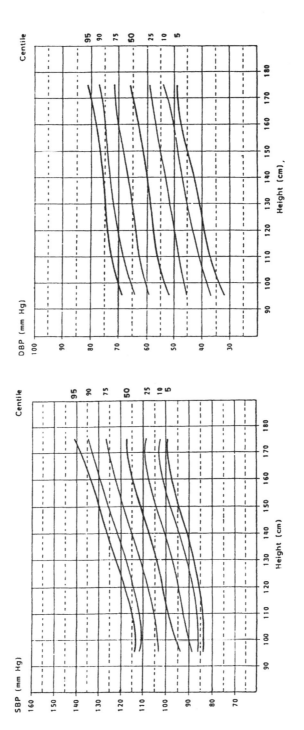

Diastolic (Korotkoff phase V)

Systolic (Korotkoff phase I)

IV NORMAL VALUES

Clinical chemistry
- Local laboratory normal ranges may be different from the values stated
- Amend figures where needed
- B = whole blood
- S = serum
- P = plasma
- N = neonatal values are different

Blood

Alkaline phosphatase: S
- Wide variation with age and laboratories
- Consult local data

Bicarbonate: P
- 18–26 mmol/l

Bilirubin (total): S, N
- Under 17 µmol/l
- Should be mainly unconjugated

Calcium: S, N
- 2.25–2.75 mmol/l

Chloride: P
- 98–105 mmol/l

Creatine phosphokinase: P
- Depends on age

Creatinine: P
- 35–105 µmol/l

Cholesterol (fasting): P
- 2.6–5.7 mmol/l

Ferritin: S
- 20–300 µg/l

Glucose (fasting): P, N
- 3–5 mmol/l

Iron: S
- 9–27 µmol/l

Lead: B
- Less than 1.75 µmol/l

Phosphate: P, N
- < 1 month 1.2–2.8 mmol/l
- > 1 month 1.3–1.8 mmol/l

Potassium: P, N
- < 1 month 3.0–6.6 mmol/l
- > 1 month 3.0–5.6 mmol/l

Protein: S
- Total 52–78 g/l
- Albumin 35–45 g/l

Sodium: P
- 135–145 mmol/l

Transferrin: S
- 2.5–4.5 g/l

Urea: P
- 2.5–6.5 mmol/l

Urinanalyis (Stix tests)
- Very sensitive
- Traces of protein or blood often a normal finding
- Presence of glucose needs further investigation

Haematology
Red cells

	Hb (g/100 ml)	MCV
4 weeks – 3 months	11–16	100–120
3–12 months	10–12.5	80–96
1–5 years	10.5–13	80–96
5–10 years	11–14	80–96
10+ years	11.5–14.5	80–96

Haemoglobin A2	<3% after 1 year
Fetal haemoglobin	<2% after 1 year
Electrophoresis	HbA only after 1 year
Platelets:	150–450 x 10⁹/l

White cells

Count	6000–15 000 x 10³/l
Neutrophils	32–52%
Lymphocytes	30–50%
Monocytes	2–10%
Eosinophils	1–6%
Basophils	<1%

Blood film
- Red cells
  — Only a few microcytes, target cells, or
  — Spherocytes and no burr cells or sickle cells
- White cells
  — No atypical cells

Serum folate: 3–20 ng/ml
Red cell folate: 100–640 ng/ml
Serum B$_{12}$: 150–1000 ng/l

Microbiology

Urine
- Microscopy: <5 cells
- No organisms
- Culture
  — Infection if pure growth + pyuria (greater than five white cells per high power field or 10 white cells per cc)
  — Mixed growth suggests a contaminated specimen

Swabs
- Commonly available swabs are:
  — Bacterial
  — Chlamydial (special transport medium)
  — Per-nasal for *Bordetella*
  — Most should be sent in transport medium

Faeces
- Microscopy
  — Ova, cysts and parasites, fresh stools required; specimens need to be repeated
- Culture
  — Bacterial causes of diarrhoea
- Electron microscopy
  — Viral causes of diarrhoea

V COLLECTING SPECIMENS

Suggest filling in the table depending on local laboratory's needs.

Blood test	Type of bottle (i.e. EDTA)	Minimum volume of blood
FBC		
ESR		
Electrolytes/creat/urea		
LFT		
TFT		
Ferritin		
Immunology (i.e. antireticulin antibodies)		

VI A LIMITED FORMULARY FOR USE IN A CHILD HEALTH CLINIC

- Children seen in child health surveillance clinics have a variety of minor problems which can be usefully treated with medications available 'on site' in the form of a small dispensary
- As the nature of community paediatric work changes from surveillance to referral work, it is useful to have at your disposal a range of medications which may need demonstration to child and parent, e.g. inhaler devices, nasal sprays and drops, creams

- Drugs should be carefully stored and maintained by a pharmacy service
- Any medications dispensed should be appropriately labelled with the child's name and clear instructions on administration
- The GP should always be informed if medications are given out at the clinic
- Acutely ill children should be discouraged from coming to a 'well baby' clinic but it is not uncommon for a sibling to require treatment on the same occasion that the healthy child is being reviewed
- Below is a list of drugs found useful in our local clinics. The list is not exhaustive but given as an example – a very small number of medicines, chosen with care, can meet a very large range of needs

Amoxycillin or other antibiotic	— for tonsillitis, otitis media
Aqueous cream	— for dry skin
Arachis oil ear drops	— removal of wax to permit inspection of tympanic membranes
Carobel	— thicken feeds
Cradocap shampoo	— for cradle cap
Chloramphenicol eye ointment 1%	— conjunctivitis
Chloramphenicol eye drops 0.5%	— conjunctivitis
Chlorpheniramine syrup 2 mg/5 ml	— allergic conditions, pruritus
Chlortetracycline cream	— impetigo
Clobetasone butyrate 0.05% cream and ointment (Eumovate)	— eczema and other skin conditions
Crotamiton lotion (Eurax)	— useful antipruritic to use after treatment for scabies and in other conditions where scratching is a major problem
Docusate sodium syrup	— constipation
Econazole cream	— ringworm
Emulsifying ointment	— for dry skin
	— also for use instead of soap in eczema
Erythromycin syrup	— severe impetigo and for children in whom penicillin is contraindicated

Glucose electrolyte solution	— gastroenteritis
Hydrocortisone 1% cream or ointment	— eczema and other skin conditions
Lactulose	— stool softener for constipation
Malathion lotion	— pediculosis (alternated with carbaryl)
Nystatin cream	— monilial napkin rash
Nystatin HC ointment	— mixed monilial/ammoniacal rashes
Nystatin oral suspension	— oral monilia
Oilatum emollient	— dry and itching skin, added to bath water
Paracetamol	— pyrexia, analgesia
Permethrin (Lyclear)	— scabies
Pseudoephedrine elixir (Sudafed)	— blocked noses in older children
Salbutamol	— asthma
Senakot syrup	— constipation
Silver nitrate sticks	— umbilical granuloma
Sytron	— iron deficiency
Trimeprazine tartrate syrup 30 mg/5 ml (Vallergan)	— hypnotic/sleep problems
Xylometazoline nasal drops	— blocked noses in babies

- Other items of use:
    - Multistix GP — for urinalysis and detection of leucocytes and nitrites in urine (UTIs)
    - Emla cream — topical anaesthetic for venepuncture
    - Vitamin drops — usually sold in clinic and recommended for all children in the first 5 years

VII IMMIGRANTS

- Technically, a bad term; may be first, second, third or later generation; term here used to identify people who have specific health risks, e.g. sickle-cell anaemia or cultural or religious practices of relevance to community paediatrics

- 1991 census
  - 8% of child population under 16 years, 1.3 million from ethnic minority group
- Largest group is Indian (2.1% of all children)
- Variation around UK large and important for community paediatrician to be aware of make up of community case load. Locality profiles are useful
- Caribbean children are more likely to live with a lone parent and have fewer siblings
- Bangladeshi and Pakistani children have more siblings; grandparents less likely to be in the UK
- Proportion of children living with one parent:
  - Caribbean   49%
  - White   15%
  - Indian, Pakistani, Bangladeshi   10%
- Of ethnic minority population aged less than 25 years, 80% born in UK
- Congenital malformations and biochemical diseases are more common in Asian families – partly as result of consanguinity (first cousin marriages)
- Infant mortality by mother's country of birth, per 1000 live births:
  - Pakistan   14.2
  - Caribbean   12.6
  - Rest of Africa   9.9
  - East Africa   7.6
  - UK   7.5
  - India   7.4
  - Bangladesh   5.5
- Sudden infant death syndrome (SIDS) is less common in Indian, Pakistani, Bangladeshi and African babies
- Experience working with different ethnic minority groups highlights the importance of different belief systems and customs which are of relevance in explaining conditions and advising about nutrition and medications

Main groups of immigrants

Group	Main countries of birth or origin	Religions
West Indian	West Indies Majority now born in UK	Christian Rastafarian
Asian	India	Hinduism, Sikhism Muslim
	Pakistan	Muslim
	Bangladesh	Muslim
	East Africa	Hinduism, Sikhism Muslim
	Sri Lanka; increasing numbers born in UK	Hinduism, Muslim, Buddhism
African	African continent	Christian, Muslim + other religions
Oriental	Hong Kong Vietnam	Buddhism Buddhism
Arab	Middle East	Muslim
S. European	Cyprus Italy Greece most born in UK	Christian Christian Christian

Health characteristics of some immigrant groups

	W. Indian	Asian	African	Oriental	Arab	S. Europe
Thalassaemia	0	+	0	0	+	+
Sickle-cell	+	0	+	0	0	0
Iron deficiency	R	++	0	0	0	0
Rickets	R	+	0	0	0	0
Tuberculosis	0	+	0	+	0	0
Congenital anomalies	0	+	0	0	+	0
Traditional healers	+	++	+	+	+	0
Different growth parameters	+	+	0	0	0	0

R = applies only to Rastafarians.

Important dietary restrictions and problems

Group	Dietary restrictions
Rastafarian	Most vegetarian – strict vegan if orthodox Avoid pork Some refuse products of the vine (grapes, raisins, wine)
Hindu	Many vegetarian No beef Many teetotal
Muslim	Avoid pork All other meat has to be correctly prepared (halal)
Sikh	Many avoid beef Many teetotal

The strictness of application of these restrictions will vary from family to family.

VIII PRACTICAL TECHNIQUES

Venepuncture

- Increasing numbers of investigations are being performed in community clinics. The first paragraph (organization of service) is relevant to doctors establishing this service for the first time

Organization of service – basic requirements

Doctors
- Doctors competent and willing to take blood with no objections from other staff, i.e. health visitors

Time
- Sufficient time between patients or before clinic to take blood. Leave 15 minutes. Labelling of bottles/form filling and difficult veins all add up!

Transport
- Use existing transport if possible. Helpful secretaries and clerks may not be covered by their insurance to transport 'bodily fluids'. This may apply to community health mail vans in some parts of the country
- Check the time the transport leaves clinic as samples left overnight may haemolyse. Try to arrange for venepunctures well before transport leaves

Equipment
- Ensure regular supplies of
  — Blue (23G) butterflies
  — Blue (23G) needles
  — Cotton wool
  — Relevant sample bottles
  — Syringes and plasters
  — Request forms

Results
- You are medico-legally liable for any investigations ordered
- Suggest keeping a *single* diary with the name/date of birth/investigations ordered and date sample taken. This allows you to chase results which have gone astray
- Contact the laboratories and speak to the Senior Chief MLSO to establish *minimum* volumes of blood needed for testing and to ensure results can be sent to *you directly*. This avoids GPs being billed if you share the same address, or results going to a secretary who is unsure which doctor within a team performed the test as it was done in another clinic

Technique
- Ensure warm peripheries. Cold hands/feet with peripheral venous shut down can be warmed with warm (not hot) towels. Ask parents to do this in waiting room

- EMLA (topical anaestheric for use over one year of age) gel is expensive but is effective if left on the skin for 60 minutes prior to venesection
- Ask for an assistant if possible
- Be aware of *minimum* blood volume needed in case of difficult venesection

Hints
- Toddlers can be distracted by toys or 'soap bubbles'
- In difficult venesections, the great saphenous is invariably present

Finger prick
- Advantage of minimal/no pain *if used with spring-loaded device* (i.e. autolet/soft touch)
- Need warm peripheries ideally
- Only obtain small volumes of blood (ideal for FBC)
- May haemolyse blood so serum potassium may be inaccurate

Technique
- Load device and ensure it works beforehand!
- Warm periphery – finger/heel
- Can smear thin layer of Vaseline on skin to help blood pool into droplets
- Keep shaking the bottle after collecting each drop of blood so as to mix with anticoagulant. Frustrating if it clots

Skin scraping
- Useful for determining fungal infection
- Need
  - Scalpel blade
  - Black blotting paper (ideally, as easier to see quantity of skin collected). Discuss with local microbiology lab

Technique
- Gently scrape affected skin, and let the loose scales fall onto the blotting paper. Small quantity needed
- Fold paper on all sides so scales can't fall out
- Send to lab with request form

Auriscope
Technique
- Use left hand for viewing child's right ear and right hand to hold auriscope for the child's left ear. Hold auriscope as you would a pen
- Pull pinna back if infant and 'up and out' if older – see Figure 5.24

Blood pressure
Technique
- Use Korotkoff phase I (systolic) and V (when pulse vanishes)
- Appropriate cuff size
- Results should be compared to height centiles

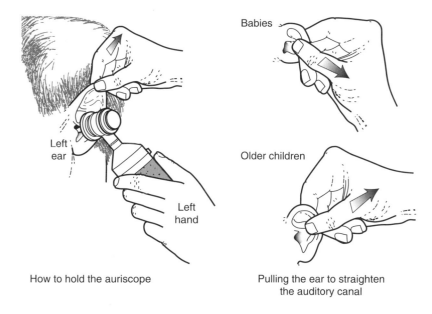

Babies

Older children

Left
ear

Left
hand

How to hold the auriscope

Pulling the ear to straighten
the auditory canal

Fig. 5.24 How to hold the auriscope.

Urine collection

Methods

Bag urine

- Use in children who haven't been potty trained. Disadvantage of possible skin contaminants
- Hint – put the bag on just before a feed. They generally micturate within 2 hours of a feed. Try to remove bag as soon as possible after collection to minimize leakage, contamination by stools and sore areas

Clean-catch

- Less danger of contamination but time-consuming
- Ensure that the toddler doesn't play with the urine collection bottle as they may again contaminate it

Catheter specimen

- Unlikely to be performed in community unless child usually uses one, i.e. spina bifida and intermittent catheterization

Supra-pubic aspiration

- Rarely done in community but no contamination if performed aseptically. Useful if repeated contaminated/equivocal bag urine samples and clean-catch failed. Need to be competent in supra-pubic aspirations

IX EXAMINATION OF TONSILS

- Examination of the tonsils can be distressing for very young children – consider whether the examination is really necessary
- If uncertain whether or not the child will tolerate the examination, he should be held by an assistant. The parent may not be the most appropriate person to do this

Correct technique is important so as to minimize distress and make the procedure as quick and effective as possible:
- Child should be sitting on assistant's lap, facing examiner
- Assistant should put one arm right around child's body, holding both child's arms down
- Assistant's other hand should hold child's forehead
- Child should be held firmly against assistant's body
  - See Figure 5.25
- Suitable light source will be required, e.g. pen-torch. Light should be bright and as even as possible
- Older children may put their tongue out or say 'ah' in order for tonsils to be visualized, otherwise tongue depressor will be required
  - Wooden in preference to metal as this may be cold
  - Do not use tongue depressor when there is a risk of acute epiglottotis as danger of obstruction

Features to look for
- Tonsils
  - Size
  - Symmetry
  - Fibrosis – due to repeated infection
  - Inflammation
  - Crypts – debris, pus
  - Exudate
  - Membrane
- Peritonsillar swelling/abscess (quinsy)
- Posterior pharyngeal wall
  - Swelling
  - Inflammation
  - Lymphoid tissue enlargement
  - Post nasal discharge
- Faucial pillars
  - Inflammation – flush on anterior pillars may indicate recurrent tonsillitis
- Uvula
  - Symmetry
  - ?Bifid – examine for submucous cleft
  - Oedema/inflammation
- Teeth
  - General condition
- Palpate cervical/submandibular glands

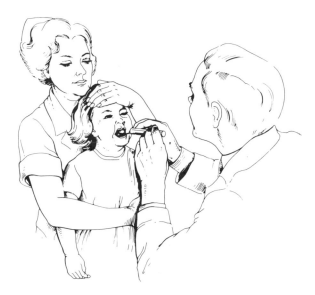

Fig. 5.25 Examining the mouth – uncooperative child.

Indications for referral for tonsillectomy
- Recurrent tonsillitis – consider:
  - Frequency of attacks
  - Severity and length of episodes
  - Time off school
  - Does the amount of illness and time off school justify removal?
- Peritonsillar abscess (quinsy) and abscess of retropharyngeal or lateral pharyngeal spaces
- Sleep apnoea syndrome – assess from history, size is not important
  - Noisy breathing in night (may sound different to ordinary snoring)
  - Periods of apnoea may be noticed by parents – can be quite prolonged
  - Child may be drowsy in daytime and perform badly at school due to poor quality of sleep
  - May be dangerous or even fatal

IX LOCALITY CHILD HEALTH PROFILING

Below are the sort of data which might be collected for a particular locality. An asterisk (*) by a particular item denotes that it is collected and used by health visitors in their caseload profiles; other items are collected at electoral ward level derived from census data or from hospital or other information sources. How many of these data are available to you? Fill in the table for two contrasting areas of your District or Health Board.

	Area 1	Area 2
Number of children < 15 years of age		
Birth rate		
% Low birth weight (< 2.5 kg)*		
Abortion rate (annual per 1000 women 15–44 years)		
Hospital admission rate (0–14 years)		
Injury and poisoning (standardized, all ages, 3 year averages)		
Rates of accidents requiring hospital treatment*		
Jarman score		
Townsend score		
% Unemployment		
% Children <5 years*		
% Family head from New Commonwealth and Pakistan*		
% Changed address*		
% Overcrowded		
% Single parents*		
% Social class V		
% Children on special needs/disability register*		
% Children on child protection register*		
% Receiving free school meals (ESMT)		
Paediatric OPD DNA rate (medical)		
Paediatric OPD DNA rate (surgical)		
% Children receiving special educational support		
% Attending a child-development centre or DHT		
% Attending social services day nurseries		
% Receiving nursery school education		
% Pre-school child care places		
Alcohol/drug abuse facility usage rate		
% Teenage pregnancy rate		
% Born to mothers <17 years*		
% Born to mothers 17–19 years*		
% Mothers smoking*		
% Receiving income support*		
Breast feeding rate at birth*		
Birth/6 week check breast feeding ratio*		
Coverage of surveillance at 8 months*		
Coverage of surveillance at 18 months*		
Completion of immunization at 24 months*		
Completion of immunization at 5 years*		
General school attendance rate		
School exclusion rate		

XI HEALTH SURVEILLANCE PROGRAMME

Age	Screening procedures	Immunization	Health education	Accident prevention
Neonate	Weight, HC (care in interpretation) Full physical examination Hips Eyes – red reflex Hearing – OAE/BSAER Heel prick tests	BCG (high risk) Hepatitis B (if mother a carrier)	Limitations of screening tests Sleeping position Smoking cessation Nutrition, baby care, sibling management, crying and sleeping problems	Bathing Falls off table Car transport
10–14 Days	Guided by results of neonatal check, jaundice, postnatal depression		Nutrition, breast feeding support, coping with baby blues	Bath-time safety
6–8 Weeks	Weight, HC, length Full examination Hips Eyes – red reflex, squint Assess risk factors for hearing and visual impairment		Early development — social behaviour — vision, hearing Family problems Depression Contraception Immunization Recognition of early illness, simple treatment for fever	Preparation for increased mobility Stairgate Fireguard
2 Months		DT Per/Polio/Hib	Immunization advice (site of injection)	
3 Months	Hips (abduction)	DT Per/Polio/Hib	Early language and social development	Scalds Glass doors
4 Months		DT Per/Polio/Hib		Window catches Car seats Bath safety
6–9 Months	Discussion of developmental progress with parents Weight, length and OFC plotted (allow for prematurity) Hips Distraction hearing test Squint		Dental prophylaxis Developmental stimulation Avoidance of sunburn	Choking, scalds and burns
12–15 Months	Check that heart and testes checks have been carried out in past reviews or arrange opportunistically	MMR	Diet, prevention of iron-deficiency anaemia Dentist Language and speech developmental stimulation	Falls from height Ponds and pools Medicines, domestic poisons
18–24 Months	Observe gait Review of development with parents Height (formal review or opportunistic) - plot Squint		Nursery, playgroup Behaviour problems, expectations Developmental guidance for language and play	Chemicals Scalds Windows Introduce awareness of road safety

BSAER = brainstem auditory evoked response; OAE = otoacoustic emissions.
Results should be recorded in the parent-held record (if used) for use by the individual clinic, and copies for the District Health Authority.

Age	Screening procedure	Immunization	Health education	Accident prevention
39–42 Months	Is this a child with special needs – consider referral to education authority Review of development speech and language, hearing, vision, behaviour with parents		School readiness Special educational needs Learning Language development Play Behaviour problems Nutrition Teeth	Garden gates Ponds and pools Road safety awareness Car seats Fires
5 Years	School entrant review	DT Per/Polio	Immunization Adjustment to school	Road safety Stranger
Year 1	Height and weight ? Heart, testes Visual acuity Hearing (sweep test) Selective follow-up of children with special needs			
7–8 Years	School nurse health appraisal Visual acuity			Road safety
Year 3	(Height)			
11–12 Years	School nurse health appraisal Visual acuity	Rubella (girls) BCG	Health education in school Teenage counselling	
Year 7	Colour vision			
14 Years	School nurse health appraisal		Careers advice Self referrals to school doctor or nurse	
16 Years		DT/Polio		

INDEX

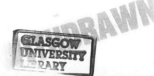